T0301080

About the authors

Beauty journalist Samantha Silver and fashion stylist Gemma Rose Breger are the expert duo behind This is Mothership, a unique fashion, beauty and lifestyle destination for time-pressed women who want to look and be their best. After climbing the ladders of the cut-throat beauty and fashion industries in London and New York, they teamed up to create a platform where they could share their wide knowledge base, as well as their own life experiences and time-saving hacks. This book is a treasury of all the tips, tricks and life hacks that Sam and Gemma have learned over the years, both as industry experts and as busy, time-pressed mums.

Sam is an award-winning beauty journalist with twenty years' experience in the beauty industry. She was beauty director at bestselling women's magazine *Stylist* for seven years before going freelance. With an impressive little black book of contacts, there is no beauty expert she hasn't interviewed. Samantha has written for *Sunday Times Style*, *Grazia*, *Glamour* and *Vogue*, been profiled in *The New York Times* and consulted for global beauty brands such as L'Oreal, GHD, Pantene and Boots.

Gemma is a fashion and celebrity stylist. Originally from Scotland, Gemma began her career in New York, working in fashion PR. Returning to the UK to live in London, she worked for Topshop for six years as a stylist and helped launch their styling service in the US. She then went freelance, styling for various celebrities, brands, magazines and TV shows, including Britney Spears, Fearne Cotton, Frankie Bridge, Joanna Lumley, *Glamour*, *Hello*, Net-a-Porter, Marks & Spencer, ASOS and *The X Factor* amongst others.

this is BEAUTY.
this is FASHION.
this is LIFE.

this is
MOTHERSHIP.

Samantha Silver & Gemma Rose Breger

PIATKUS

PIATKUS

First published in Great Britain in 2024 by Piatkus

1 3 5 7 9 10 8 6 4 2

Copyright © Gemma Breger and Sam Silver 2024

The moral right of the authors has been asserted.

All rights reserved. No part of this publication may be reproduced,
stored in a retrieval system, or transmitted in any form or by any means,
without the prior permission in writing of the publisher, nor be otherwise
circulated in any form of binding or cover other than that in which it is published
and without a similar condition including this condition being imposed
on the subsequent purchaser.

A CIP catalogue record for this book is available from the British Library.

ISBN 978-0-349-44017-0

Illustrations on pages 6, 38, 66, 97, 98, 114, 115, 121, 133, 135, 152, 156, 176, 190, 209 and 232
by Attabeira German de Turowski;
illustrations on pages 10, 14, 29, 30 45, 48, 51, 52, 64, 76 and 165 by Liane Payne;
all photographs authors' own.

Designed and set by EM&EN

Printed and bound in Great Britain by Clays Ltd, Elcograf S.p.A.

Papers used by Piatkus are from well-managed forests
and other responsible sources.

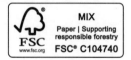

PIATKUS
An imprint of
Little, Brown Book Group
Carmelite House
50 Victoria Embankment
London EC4Y 0DZ
An Hachette UK Company

www.hachette.co.uk
www.littlebrown.co.uk

NOTE: product prices are given to help the reader identify a specific product and are based on
those available when the book went into production in February 2024.

To all who have joined us on board the Mothership,

this book is for you.

contents

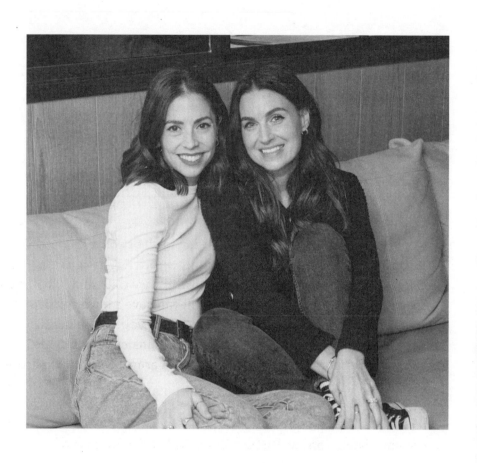

introduction

If you're reading this book because you follow us on Instagram (@thisismothership) then, hello! If you're new around here, then hi, it's so great to meet you – and welcome aboard the Mothership. In 2016, we left behind our careers in fashion and beauty, working on TV and magazines, and created our own platform, which would go on to become your online oracle for all things fashion, beauty and lifestyle. We know how hard it is to juggle a busy social life, job, friends and family while still making time for yourself, but we also think it's pretty important to do so. Looking after yourself can have a huge positive impact on your well-being, so we're here to help you streamline all aspects of your life, so you can think clearly. Think of us as a duo of experts in your pocket; a mini magazine team armed with the expertise to see you through your busy day.

Instagram is packed with beauty tips, fashion hacks and lifestyle advice, and offers everyone a space to show off their skills, give their recommendations and share their opinions. But an overload of information isn't always a good thing – too many opinions can become confusing, and not everyone is an expert. The dress that suits one person may not suit you. What transforms someone else's skin may not transform yours. And it's important to recognise that it's very rare for a product or technique to truly live up to Insta-hype.

We're coming from a place of expertise. We've both lived, breathed and slept our industries from the age of eighteen (professionally, at least – our fascination started long before). We have worked so hard for the qualifications, the degrees, and the experience we've gained working on magazines and behind the scenes on television shows. This means we can really back up everything that we tell you. And we won't just tell you what works for us – we can tell you what will work for *you*, how it will work and why.

One of the loveliest things about being on social media is the immediate feedback that we get from our followers. Our hearts genuinely lift when a message arrives in our inbox to tell us that one of our recommendations has positively changed someone's day, making their lives run a little more smoothly, or given them a much-needed confidence boost, even in the smallest of ways. We feel honoured to have grown such a warm, sensitive and supportive community, and we will always be grateful for that.

We hope that in this book, we can demystify some of the 'rules' set in place by women's magazines over the years, simplifying your routines so you can get on with the most important things and make the most of your day.

Before we get started, you probably want to know a little bit more about us, so let us introduce ourselves.

Meet Sam, aka the Beauty Expert

'The beauty industry is in my genes.'

Hello, I'm Sam. Before *This is Mothership* began, I was a beauty journalist. You might have read my work in magazines like *Stylist*, *Grazia*, *Glamour* and *Sunday Times Style*. I won awards for my writing, travelled across the world and saw behind the glossy scenes of the beauty industry. There isn't a beauty expert, top make-up artist or household-name hairdresser that I haven't interviewed. I spent over a decade working with experts, getting up close and personal over the make-up table backstage at Fashion Week, and speaking to scientists on lab visits.

But let's rewind further. Before any of that, I was born into the beauty world. I grew up in Sheffield, and spent much of my childhood in my mum's beauty salons. I folded treatment menus, restocked cotton wool and eventually, aged fifteen, I landed myself a job on the reception desk. This 'on the ground' training ignited an interest in the world of beauty, and showed me first-hand how transformative beauty could be for the women who walked through those doors.

Some of my earliest memories are of playing at my grandma's dressing table, painting my nails with her Mavala nail polishes (tiny little doll-sized bottles of pinks and reds) and spraying her fancy cut-glass perfume diffusers with those big squeezy balls at the end. When I slept over, I was allowed to wash my hair with her Kerastase shampoo; those orange bottles with the French writing on seemed so sophisticated. Even as my grandma got older and her memory left her, she still had her nails painted and went for a weekly blow-dry. She always looked immaculate.

All in all, it seemed to be fate that while on a summer internship at *Glamour* magazine in 2001, I discovered this thing called 'the beauty cupboard': an Aladdin's cave, heaving with skincare, make-up, hair products, fake tan, fancy shower gels and fragrances. I discovered, to my amazement, that people were actually *paid* to try out beauty products and treatments, and then write about them. There was no looking back after that. Over a decade later, with a slew of titles under my belt, nine industry awards to my name and a little black contacts book filled to the brim with the who's who of the beauty world, I did something no one thought I would do. I tossed it all in.

I still produce beauty content, but now I do it online, direct to our This is Mothership audience. And here, on these pages, I'm excited to untangle the complicated cacophony of beauty rules and ideals with which we're inundated on a daily basis, and simplify everything, sharing straightforward beauty advice for all ages, skin tones, skin types and budgets.

Because I believe that when used properly, the beauty world and all it has to offer can be truly life-affirming, mind-altering and mood-boosting.

Meet Gemma, aka the Fashion Expert

'Fashion is in my blood.'

I grew up with two grandmas, each of whom was exceptionally cool in her own way. Every time I saw them, they were both meticulously dressed, and I'm sure this is where my love of fashion began.

My Grandma Ann (my mum's mum) was a huge monochrome lover. She had a wardrobe full of black and white, punctuated with little pops of colour (often in the form of her bold lipstick.) She knew exactly how to dress for her shape, and doing so was important to her. She lived in Canada but she visited us often, and we visited her. I can still remember sitting on the edge of the bed in our spare room while she unpacked. She would always explain to me how every item had to have its own compartment (no prizes for guessing where my obsession with organisation comes from!), and she showed me how she had planned all her outfits for every day of the trip, down to the jewellery. Every piece could be mixed and matched with another, and the shoes were carefully selected to work with as many outfits as possible. She knew what she was doing, and she did it so well. She passed away in 2021, but my memories of her are so fond, and her packing tips will be ingrained in me for ever!

My Grandma Ida (my dad's mum) is ninety-seven and lives in Glasgow. To this day, she's one of the coolest people I know. Her outfits are wild and her style has always been really creative; she never sticks to trends, she just wears what she loves. From dressing in leather trousers and baker-boy caps when picking me up from school, to modelling matching co-ords in the form of a floral trench with matching hat and skirt, she always stands out. She epitomises elegance, and has no idea just how fashionable she is. She talks now about how unimportant other people's opinions of her outfits are; all that matters is that she likes them. I love this attitude, and I'm sure it had a big impact on me growing up.

I've been in the world of fashion professionally for almost twenty years and have seen it from all angles. I began my career studying fashion communication and marketing (with a side of psychology) at the University of Leeds, before spending time in New York, where I worked at New York Fashion Week and for two different fashion PRs: one at an agency, and one at the Ted Baker head office. It was here that I learned PR wasn't creative enough for me. I came home from New York and moved to London, where I began working as a stylist for Topshop. I stayed there for six years, and in 2009 I helped with the launch of their styling services at the first-ever US Topshop in New York. After this adventure, I left to become a freelance fashion stylist, which involved working for TV shows like *The X Factor* and *Britain's Next Top Model*, and magazines such as *Glamour*, *Hello!* and *Grazia*. I worked with many A-list celebrities (if only I could share *those* stories!) and ultimately went on to create This is Mothership.

I've learned so much on this journey, and want to share with you all the tips and tricks I've discovered. I'm going to teach you how to be wiser with what you buy, how to wear it and how to make it last. This isn't just about learning to dress better, it's about learning to feel better about yourself, because I believe that fashion is about so much more than just some clothes hanging in your wardrobe.

So, without further ado, let's get started.

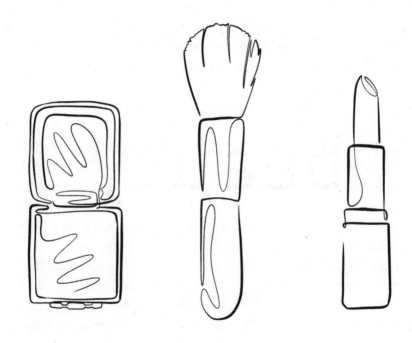

- part one -

beauty

...

Beauty is often seen as frivolous. An added extra. A vanity project. There is sometimes the presumption that a person must have a lot of time on their hands to be able to indulge in it. As women, we often feel guilty for spending time on ourselves. We might struggle to take time away from our desks, instead eating lunch as we frantically type, and we often find it almost impossible to prioritise time for ourselves over our friends and family.

However, as we will explore together on these pages, beauty is far from frivolous; in fact, spending a little time on beauty can contribute towards women's positive mental health and confidence.

Over the years, beauty has become complicated, with multi-step routines and social media feeds filled with this 'must-have' or that 'next-big-thing'. The noise can often become too much, not to mention the increasing cost of investing in one beauty product after the next.

I know how busy you are, and that you may not have the brain space to read up on the latest 'how, what and why' when it comes to your beauty regime – so I'm laying it all out here for you. Education is key, so I've given you all the top-line skincare science to help you make your own informed choices, alongside the backstage tips and make-up tricks that I have learned by interviewing every pro make-up artist over two decades. There's even a chapter that will give you the best hair of your life, every day of the week. And just so that we're clear on the 'beauty is not frivolous' front, I'm also going to get serious, sharing my personal experience of medically diagnosed burnout and how the beauty industry saved me.

My goal for this section is to help you prioritise, simplify and find a routine that works for you and your lifestyle, without compromising on feeling like *you*. I've got you.

Sam x

- 1 -

simplifying skincare

Skincare can be overwhelmingly confusing. There's so much being sold to us these days, and so much we seemingly should be using. Do we need to double-cleanse? Do we need a serum? What about eye cream? How about retinol? And what about that ten-step Korean skincare routine – should we be doing that?

We all have enough on our plates without adding a million unnecessary, expensive (and, quite frankly, skin-clogging) steps into the morning rush, so in this chapter I'm going to break it all down for you, explaining what each product is, where it goes and what it does.

There is real power in feeling happy with your skin. I know that when my skin is looking good, I'm able to look people in the eye when I'm speaking to them and I feel more confident. When my skin is looking bad, I want to hide away.

About Your Skin

Your skin is the biggest organ of your body. We take it for granted, but it does so many different things on the daily. I'm going to explain a bit about how the science behind the skin works, so you will know how skincare ingredients work on *it*. If you're educated on how the skin works, you'll be able to see through some of the marketing claims that certain brands make. Here comes the science bit . . .

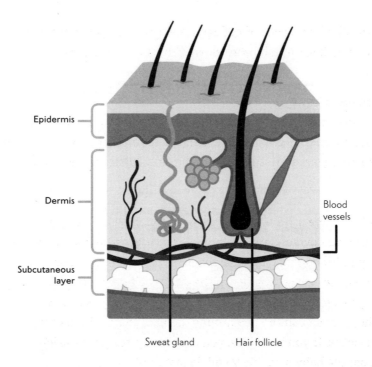

Epidermis

Dermis

Subcutaneous layer

Blood vessels

Sweat gland　　Hair follicle

The epidermis

This is the outermost layer of skin. It's the part you can see. It's constantly renewing. New cells are made lower down, and travel to the top over the course of a month. These then replace the cells that sit on the surface and have got duller over time. As we get older, the shedding of these dead, dull cells slows down, which is why we don't look as 'glowy' and why we may need to introduce exfoliants to remove them (more on that later). Topical skincare products will only ever treat the epidermis; anything deeper needs a needle. Any product that claims to 'sink' beneath the skin's surface is selling you a dream.

The dermis

This contains your blood vessels and nerves, as well as collagen and elastin, which give skin its bounce and ability to snap back. The dermis is also home to your skin's natural stores of hyaluronic acid. If you tug at your skin when you're younger, it 'snaps back' instantly, but as we age, and the skin's reserves of collagen, elastin and hyaluronic acid deplete, it sinks back much more slowly. This is when wrinkles and dry skin form.

Subcutaneous tissue

This helps provide insulation, regulate temperature and store fat. Because subcutaneous tissue is the deepest layer of the skin, it attaches the other skin layers to tissues under the skin, like bones and muscles.

★ **TIM TIP:** There are a few rules we need to follow if we're going to be experts on how to look after our own skin, and the first one is: no face wipes! When I met Gemma, the first thing I changed about her beauty regime was getting her to the ditch the face wipes. Not only are they bad for the planet, but they also don't really cleanse your face; they just smush the dirt around. Replace them with flannels or muslin cloths. If you have kids, you may have a few of these left over from the baby days. They will do just fine.

How to Build Your AM/PM Routines

One of the most common requests I receive is to show my AM and PM skincare routines on Instagram. A good skincare routine is one that's realistic for your lifestyle. Make it too fancy, and you'll never stick to it. Everyone's routine will look a little different depending on how much time they have, as well as their own skin concerns and skin type, but these are the basic principles of a skincare routine . . .

AM routine

The main point of your AM routine is to set yourself (and your skin) up for the day and protect it from the outside world: pollution, sun and environmental aggressors all contribute to the quality of your skin. There are three fundamentals: cleanse, hydrate and protect. Within those categories there are many steps you can take – which is why so many people get confused – but if you are *really* short on time in the mornings, the basics are cleanse, hydrate, eye cream, SPF. The rest can be saved until the evening. Off you go.

(Note that these are the steps to follow – I'll look at the products themselves in detail throughout the chapter.)

Cleanse

This is non-negotiable. A quick, non-foaming cleanse to ready your skin for the day ahead and remove any sweat or product residue that's built up overnight. Remove it with a damp flannel or muslin.

> ★ **TIM TIP:** Don't cleanse your face in the shower. It's likely that the water will be too hot for the delicate skin on your face, and this could strip the skin, damaging it and causing it to become dry or dehydrated. Cleanse before or after you get into the shower, with warm water.

Hydrate

Next, apply hyaluronic acid (HA). HA grabs on to moisture and sucks it deep down so it should be applied to damp skin that is still slightly wet from cleansing – or you can give your face a quick spritz of a facial spray to dampen it. Apply your HA all over. (See page 19 and the glossary for more on HA.)

Eye cream

Using your ring finger (which has the least amount of pressure, meaning it won't drag the delicate skin), apply a hydrating formula around the orbital bone (use your finger to feel your way along the edges of the bone). Some eye creams have light-reflecting properties that help to diminish the look of dark circles, and some come with a depuffing, cool ceramic tip; both are useful for the mornings.

Serum/oil

Measure a couple of drops into the palm of your hand and then use your fingertips to press into the skin. If you're using a serum with vitamin C or another antioxidant, this is when to use it. If you don't have time for this step in the morning rush, that's absolutely fine.

Moisturiser

Choose one that's suitable for your skin type. Apply in sweeping, upward motions. This will lock in everything that came before it.

SPF

Always factor 50. Always two fingers' worth. Non-negotiable. SPFs are so advanced these days, they are a pleasure to use. This is the best anti-ageing product in your entire beauty arsenal. The last step before moving on to make-up.

★ **TIM TIP:** As a rule of thumb, the order of application is thinnest to thickest. This is why we go from your spritz to your serum, and/or your oil, and finally your creams.

The Perfect Dose

Do you know how much you should be using when it comes to your skincare? Chances are, you're probably using too much. Not only will this overload the skin, but it also means you're wasting money. Knowing the right amount of product to use will save you money in the long run, as your products will last longer and be more effective.

So how much product should you use?

Cleanser	Serum	Eye Cream	Moisturiser	SPF
50p piece	5p piece	Grain of rice (per eye)	20p piece	Two fingers' worth

PM routine

We usually have a bit more time in the evenings to treat our skin, but if time is tight, we have one non-negotiable here: cleanse your skin every night, *without fail*. You have been told. For me, I do it as soon as I get in from picking up my kids from school (or whatever sports activity I've been ferrying them to that evening). Some people get an 'ahhhh' moment when they get home and remove their bra; for me, that feeling comes when my face is clean after a day of commuting, sweating and stressing (none of which are good for your skin).

Double-cleanse

Ten to fifteen per cent of make-up is left on your skin after cleansing, so to get it properly clean at the end of the day, we need to get into the habit of double-cleansing, otherwise whatever you put on your skin afterwards isn't going to be able to do its job properly.

Remove any make-up first. A micellar water and cotton pad will do the job. Now is the time to remove your SPF, a cleansing oil will really take the day off, removing it with your damp muslin or flannel. Then go in for your second cleanse, giving yourself a little bit of time to really massage it in before removing with your muslin or flannel.

Active

If you're using retinol, wait until your skin is dry, then apply a pea-sized amount, two to three times a week. Wait twenty to thirty minutes before applying anything else. If you aren't using a retinol, this is when to apply your exfoliating acid – think glycolic acid (great for getting a glow), salicylic acid (for blemish-prone skin) or lactic acid (for boosting cell turnover on dehydrated or dry skin). Use every other night.

Eye cream

Again, apply using your ring finger around the orbital bone.

Serum/oil

As before, measure a couple of drops into the palm of your hand and then use your fingertips to press it into the skin.

Night cream

Apply in sweeping upward motions. Like your AM moisturiser, it will lock in everything that came before it. Ceramides (to strengthen the skin's barrier) and humectants (to lock in moisture) are good ingredients to look for in a night cream.

Spend or save?

Everyone wants to know where to spend and where to save.
My general rule of thumb is, if a product gets washed down the
drain (cleanser, shower gel, face wash) spend less on it, saving the
extra cash for the products that sit on your skin all day.

Night and Day Creams

Do you really need a separate day and night moisturiser? The answer is
yes, because they do completely different things.

Research by Estée Lauder and Cleveland University Hospital
concluded that inadequate sleep increased signs of ageing.[1] The study
found that women who regularly got less than five hours' sleep had
twice the lines and wrinkles, suffered from more dehydration and were
more vulnerable to UV damage (i.e. pigmentation) compared to those
who enjoyed seven hours of sleep or more.

So while you're up all night with your baby, struggling to sleep due
to work stress, or waiting up for a teenager to get home (delete as
appropriate), you need a really clever skincare formula that can tackle
all of this for you.

In the day . . .
. . . you need a moisturiser that will protect your skin from UV damage
(yes, even in winter). It must also act as an invisible shield – pollution,
daily grime and dirt cling to your face everywhere you turn; from the
second you leave your house, your skin is under attack. Day-specific
moisturisers are therefore designed to shield and protect your skin
from all these factors.

Whereas at night . . .

. . . you need to repair your skin. Sleep is one of the best anti-ageing ingredients. While we sleep, growth-factor hormones start to repair cell damage that happens during the day, with their work peaking during the deepest first two hours of sleep and continuing throughout the night. When you're surviving on minimal broken sleep, your skin just doesn't have enough time to repair itself. Also, the shock of being jolted awake by a screaming baby/snoring partner/bed-hopping child triggers spikes in cortisol, the stress hormone, leading to puffiness, inflammation and collagen breakdown, which means skin stops being as firm and plump as it was in our twenties. Ugh. This is why it's so important that our night-time moisturiser works double-duty overnight.

M&S Formula Sleep & Replenish Ultimate Sleep Cream, £23
I swear this is one of my most-loved beauty products. It's one of the beauty industry's best-kept secrets. It feels heavenly to apply, and leaves your skin feeling silky soft and looking radiant the next morning. It's known as 'eight hours' sleep in a pot' thanks to its remarkable ability to basically recharge your skin's batteries.

Caudalie Vinoperfect Dark Spot Correcting Glycolic Night Cream, £25
Skin pigmentation is a common issue for many people in the UK, probably due to our general lack of SPF use throughout the year. This is why so many night creams contain glycolic acid: it's the ideal overnight exfoliator. Expect to see brighter, more even-toned skin after two months. And it's vegan.

Elemis Peptide Four Plumping Pillow Facial Sleep Mask, £48
At night, body temperature rises as we go into repair and recovery mode. As a result, your skin loses hydration while you sleep. This super-cooling gel mask fights the visible signs of tired, dull skin by helping to seal in hydrating actives throughout the night, leaving your skin looking radiant, refreshed and well-rested in the morning.

Skincare Q&As

What is a serum?

A serum is an intensive, lightweight formula that can deeply penetrate the skin, as it contains molecules that are much smaller than those in a moisturiser. Look for one containing antioxidants to provide protection from environmental damage.

Why can't I use my moisturiser as an eye cream?

The skin around the eye is one tenth of the density of the skin on the face, so an eye product has to be much lighter than a moisturiser. When applying, avoid puffiness by steering clear of the tear duct.

What is an acid?

Acids – though the name might sound terrifying – are one of the easiest, fastest and most sure-fire ways to revitalise your skin and have you glowing in no time. Put simply, acids work on the superficial, top layers of the skin, dissolving and breaking down the bonds between skin, sloughing away the dull, bumpy, older skin cells, and revealing a fresher, more even surface layer. Choose from AHAs or BHAs depending on your skin's needs. Check out the glossary for more information.

What is an antioxidant?

Antioxidants are molecules that help neutralise harmful free radicals in our bodies. Free radicals are unstable atoms that can damage cells, causing signs of premature ageing, such as lines, wrinkles and pigmentation. They are triggered by things such as exposure to cigarette smoking, air pollutants, and other external aggressors.

What is the skin barrier?

The skin barrier is like a fence. It's designed to keep in some things (like moisture) while keeping out anything that can negatively affect your skin. And just like a real fence, the skin barrier can be affected and damaged by environmental factors. Once you have tears in your skin barrier, it's more likely that your skin will suffer with dryness, irritation, breakouts, etc. Keeping a healthy skin barrier is key.

Welcome to Skin School: Skincare Ingredients Everyone Over Thirty Should Use

Intrigued by beauty's most effective ingredients but don't know where to start? I bet you feel like you hear words like retinol, acid and vitamin C multiple times a day on Instagram or TV ads, but do you actually know what they do? After going through our Skin School, you'll be fully knowledgeable when it comes to reading the back of skincare products, and equipped to make the right decisions for your skin. You'll even be able to educate your friends and family.

Hyaluronic acid

Hyaluronic acid may sound intimidating – an *acid*, for your face?! No thanks. But science shows us it's one of the best ingredients you could use in skincare. Close to perfection, in fact, as it promises plumper, bouncier, more juicy-looking skin. It's gentle, loves all skin types, pairs phenomenally with other ingredients (even retinol and AHAs), and can be used in your AM and PM routines.

Hyaluronic acid is a naturally occurring gel-like substance that has the unique ability to retain moisture, keeping skin soft and supple. But we produce less and less hyaluronic acid as we age. From around the age of twenty-five the skin's own production of hyaluronic acid slowly decreases, resulting in dullness, thirsty skin, and the formation of fine lines, leading to the first wrinkles.

Hyaluronic acid holds over 1,000 times its own weight in water, so when used in skincare, it literally acts as a moisture magnet, binding water to the skin. This increases the skin's dewiness and bounciness, and plumps up those surface lines and wrinkles.

Try: L'Oréal Paris Revitalift 1.5% Hyaluronic Acid Filler Serum, £25 // Beauty Pie Triple Hyaluronic Acid Lipopeptide Serum, members £19/ non-members £85 // The Inkey List Hyaluronic Acid Serum, £8

★ **TIM TIP:** Always apply to damp skin. As a moisture magnet, hyaluronic acid will suck up any moisture sitting on the skin's surface. If applied to dry skin, it will draw moisture from its nearest source (your skin), taking what it can and thus leaving your skin drier than when you started. So apply on skin that is still lightly damp from cleansing, or use a facial mist before application.

Retinol

Retinol belongs to a family called 'retinoids', which derive from vitamin A. They improve skin turnover (which means they slough away dead, dull skin cells from the surface of the skin to reveal the newer, radiant ones), and reduce the breakdown of collagen (which means skin stays plumper for longer). They also help to reduce fine lines, pigmentation and acne marks. So, in simple terms, retinol is a one-stop-shop, anti-ageing powerhouse that we should all be using – that is, if you want plumper, radiant, even-toned skin.

There are a few retinol rules to know if you want to benefit from this pigmentation-blitzing, acne-reducing, wrinkle-banishing skincare superhero.

1. **Start LOW and SLOW**
   Introduce it gradually into your regime. Don't go for a high percentage just because you think it will work quicker.

2. **Apply in the evenings to cleansed skin**
   Start with two nights a week, slowly progressing to every other night.

3. **Add nourishing products into your skincare regime**
   Irritation, dryness and flakiness come as part of the initial package when you first start using retinol. Adding nourishing products such as a gentle, simple moisturiser or a barrier repair cream will help to counteract any of that.

4. **Use the recommended amount**
   This is usually a pea-size amount. Using more is not going to make it work quicker.

5. **Do not forget SPF**
   Retinol increases your skin's sun sensitivity, plus it will leave you with lots of fresh new skin on the surface you don't want to damage. If you're using retinol in the evening, you MUST use factor fifty in the morning.

Try: L'Oréal Paris Revitalift Laser Pure Retinol Night Serum, £13 // Medik8 Crystal Retinal 1, £45 // Dermalogica Skin Care Retinol Serum, £89

Can I use retinol when pregnant or breastfeeding?

Because to begin with, retinol can cause some skin sensitivity, redness, flaking and irritation, and because our skin often becomes temperamental when we're pre- and post-partum, experts advise that retinol shouldn't be used when pregnant or just after. This is pretty annoying, because pregnancy and early motherhood is really where the majority of our skincare concerns appear – hands up if you suffered from hyperpigmentation and melasma during your pregnancy and developed a general greige-toned, fine-lined, sleep-deprived skin appearance. Yep, us too. Plant-based extract bakuchiol has become something of an alternative in recent years; Medik8 Bakuchiol Peptides Serum (£45), is a great option here. As it's anti-inflammatory, it would also be great for those with sensitive skin or skin prone to eczema. It offers similar results to classic retinol-based products, at a slower pace.

If you're pregnant, speak to your GP at your next appointment about what ingredients you can and can't use on your skin.

Vitamin C

Vitamin C is a potent antioxidant and a great tool for brightening the skin. It can tackle hyperpigmentation, reduce redness and protect your skin from environmental aggressors. It also boosts collagen production, which makes skin plumper and firmer, and generally leaves it looking glowy and bright.

But not all vitamin Cs are born equal. The most potent is straight-up vitamin C, known as ascorbic or L-ascorbic acid (look for 10–20 per cent for real potency), but there are plenty of vitamin C derivatives, too.

Try: SkinCeuticals CE Ferulic, £94 // L'Oréal Paris Revitalift Clinical 12% Pure Vitamin C Serum, £30

★ **TIM TIP:** Apply your vitamin C product in the morning. Vitamin C is a potent antioxidant, meaning it will protect your skin from all manner of ageing aggressors like pollution and UV rays. After cleansing, apply your vitamin C, wait a few moments, and then apply your serums or moisturisers as normal. Always apply SPF; while vitamin C limits the damage caused by UV rays, it's not a sunscreen.

Ceramides

Ceramides are fatty acids that are naturally found between our skin's cells, making up 50 per cent of the skin's barrier. They retain moisture, which keeps the skin hydrated. They are essentially the glue that holds our skin cells together, keeping the skin barrier intact and healthy. A healthy skin barrier helps seal in moisture and keeps out harmful elements.

As we age, ceramide levels deplete, naturally dropping after the age of thirty. Applying them topically helps to keep skin plump and firm, and can treat sensitivity and fine lines.

Everyone over the age of thirty should be using ceramides topically to restore the levels in their skin. Ceramides are ideal for all skin types, especially if you have a compromised skin barrier – so sensitive, dry and dehydrated skin types will all benefit.

Try: CeraVe Hydrating Cleanser, £11 // La Roche-Posay Cicaplast, £18 // SkinCeuticals Epidermal Repair, £70 // Dr Jart Ceramidin Cream, £38 // Nip + Fab Ceramide Fix Serum, £29 // Dermalogica Stabilising Repair Cream, £65

Blemish Busters

Our skin goes through a lot hormonally, thanks to puberty, pregnancy (if that's your journey) and then perimenopause. Throughout these stages, we are often followed – or should I say 'plagued'? – by spots. Here's how to battle blemishes as a grown-up. Pick your fighter . . .

The cleanser: SkinCeuticals Blemish + Age Cleanser, £45
This stuff addresses my two primary concerns – acne and signs of ageing – in one fell swoop. I've found that it's ideal for keeping the smaller whiteheads and surface bumps away, and it doesn't dry out my skin whatsoever. It's been my go-to morning cleanser for the best part of six years, and has both salicylic acid and glycolic acid to smooth, lipo-hydroxy acid to decongest pores, and 2 per cent dioic acid to halt excess oil.

The pro treatment: Drunk Elephant Babyfacial, £56
I honestly can't stress enough how epic this is. A 25 per cent AHA and 2 per cent BHA blend of glycolic, salicylic, tartaric, lactic and citric acids, this supercharged concoction helps provide deep exfoliation that allows for silky-smooth skin that *really* is baby soft. After cleansing, apply a thin layer to your face, leave for twenty minutes and clean off with a flannel for an otherworldly glow. Use once a week.

The face mask: Beauty Pie Super Pore-Detox Purifying Black Clay Mask, £13 members/£45 non-members
This purifying clay mask is the master of all mud masks, giving a seriously deep pore clean in minutes. Glycolic and lactic acids deeply exfoliate, kaolin clay absorbs excess oil, while antiseptic eucalyptus oil calms and purifies skin. Great for oily T-zones or just before your period.

The targeted treatment: Murad Deep Relief Blemish Treatment, £36
Designed to blitz deep blemishes and reduce redness – keep this one in

your bathroom for emergencies. Dip a cotton bud into BHA salicylic acid, then apply it directly onto the spot – it penetrates skin to unclog pores, resulting in a reduction in blackheads, blemishes and redness overnight.

The acid: Paula's Choice 2% BHA Liquid Exfoliant, £14
A real cult product, we have gone through bottles and bottles of this over the years. When a breakout hits, this is essential. Apply the formula using a cotton pad; it tingles slightly but doesn't sting. Laced with BHA salicylic acid, it removes dead skin cells both on the skin's surface and within the pore, helping to reduce blemishes and blackheads for clear skin.

A Word on SPF

We can't not mention SPF here. After all, it is the greatest anti-ageing tool with which you could possibly arm yourself. We are of the generation that spent our twenties baking ourselves in the sun, and we have the pigmentation to prove it. Now in our thirties and armed with knowledge, we are trying to reverse the damage we did and protect our skin from any further harm.

The biggest skincare advice I can give to you is to wear SPF every day, come rain or shine. Factor 50s are now so advanced that they feel and look like skin-enhancing primers, sitting beautifully whether worn underneath make-up or alone. The best SPF is one that you want to use. It may take a little trial and error, but once you find the one, you'll actually enjoy wearing it daily.

Your SPF should be the last item of skincare you put on your face prior to make-up (if you are wearing any). If your foundation contains SPF50, it is not enough. You don't put on enough foundation on to get the adequate amount of protection. Two fingers' worth of SPF is the rule. Draw a line of SPF along your middle and index fingers; *that* is how much you should wear every day. And wear it 365 days a year, even on cloudy days.

People ask when you should start wearing SPF daily; if you are old enough to wear make-up, and have a cleansing regime, then you should be wearing SPF. You'll find our tips on SPFs in the travel section starting on page 209 and remember, SPF is a must all year round not just when travelling, even in our climate.

> ★ **TIM TIP:** There are two types of sun rays, UVA and UVB. The easy way to remember them is 'A is for ageing, B is for burning'. UVA rays are constant throughout the year, and can penetrate through glass. This is why we say you should wear SPF daily, even in winter.

The Monthly Beauty Cycle

You might be used to the odd pimple popping up when you're on your period, but do you really know how much of an impact your monthly cycle has on your skin? Once you pay attention, you'll notice a repetitive pattern and understand how to treat it accordingly. For example, you might use a clarifying serum before your period to battle those breakouts from rearing their ugly heads, then swap it out for a formula that addresses dullness once you're actually on your period.

The menstrual phase
This is your actual period, when your uterus sheds its lining.

If you're wondering why your skin might be looking dull during this time, the reason is that during your period, your oestrogen and progesterone levels fall, so body temperature and blood circulation are both lower than usual. The lack of blood circulation causes skin to appear dull, and sebum production (high at other times of your cycle) decreases, leading to dryer skin.

Combat this by using products that are high in vitamin C and antioxidants to alleviate dullness and revive your natural glow. Check out our vitamin C advice on page 22.

★ **TIM TIP:** Partial to a Haribo (or twenty) when on your period? Breakouts in the zone around your jawline are often hormonal, but they can also be worsened by sugar, which triggers insulin production, prompting an increase in hormones, leading to spots. Try to lay off the sugar when you're on your period, and see if you notice fewer spots forming. Alternatively, Consultant Dermatologist and Nutritionist Dr Thivi Maruthappu suggests swapping sweets for dark chocolate with nuts; the added fat creates less of a 'spike'.

The follicular phase
This starts on the last day of your period and ends when you start to ovulate.

This is your skin's time to shine, and the stage when it tends to be in its best condition.

During this time, simply stick to what your skin knows and loves.

The luteal phase (days 15–28)
This phase generally starts ten days before your period and happens while you're ovulating.

As we all know, the PMS phase is the one that causes the most visible changes to your skin. In the second half of the cycle, rising levels of progestogens and androgens kick our oil glands into overdrive. This attracts bacteria, which thrives and leads to oilier skin and premenstrual blemishes, typically around the chin.

Combat this by using a cleanser with salicylic acid to get rid of excess oils, and a nourishing moisturiser to rehydrate. Look for formulas containing ingredients that calm inflammation – and exfoliating properties to avoid the build-up of dead skin cells. Check out our Blemish Busters section on page 24.

> ★ **TIM TIP:** Give yourself a little lymphatic drainage before bed to reduce period puffiness, using massage to apply your night cream. This can firm muscles and flush out fluid. Bend your fingers, place your knuckles under your chin and drag them along your jawline and towards your ears. Repeat ten times on each side.

You Are Now Entering the Skincare Zone

Work out your skin type

Wash your face with a gentle cleanser, wait ten minutes and then take this test. Take a single-ply piece of tissue paper and press it all over your face. Hold it up to the light. Use the chart on the next page to work out what type of skin you have.

As a general rule, oily skin is usually characterised by enlarged pores, shine and blackheads, and is caused by the excessive production of sebum, aka oil, which keeps skin hydrated. The overproduction of oil tends to clog pores, mixing with dead skin cells and bacteria to cause breakouts. Look for the word 'noncomedogenic' on skincare products, which means that it won't clog pores further, and opt for

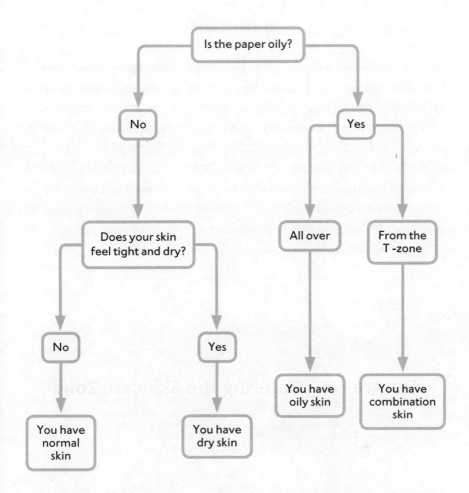

gentle cleansers that won't send skin haywire, triggering further oil production.

Dry and dehydrated skin might seem similar but they are very different. Take a look at the hydration quiz on page 33 to understand this skin type further.

Of course, many of us don't fit into either 'type', and have normal skin – or more of a combination skin, where a whole load of things are happening at once. This could be your skin's natural state, or it may be caused by 'life', which brings me to the 'zones'.

In the Zone

As a generation of women, we're very precise, whether we're choosing between a morning latte, flat white or matcha to deliver just the right caffeine hit, or deliberating over an Insta caption. When it comes to our complexions, however, we seem to have a different ethos, often using the same skincare product across our faces in the hope that what works for our oily foreheads will also hydrate our dry cheeks. It won't.

You've heard of the T-zone, but what about the rest of your face? Let's take a look at the different zones, so you can identify and target your own personal problem areas.

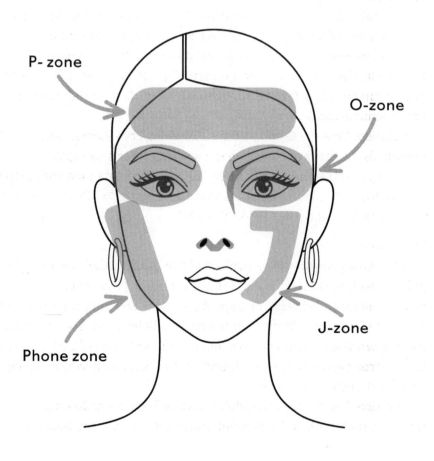

The P-zone

The top third of your forehead (the pigmentation zone) is the 'peak of your face', and the first area to be bombarded by aggressors – sun, rain and wind all hit here first. Couple that with our stingy SPF application in this area for fear of a greasy hairline, and pigmentation spots are likely to appear.

Solution: Keep a stick of SPF (they look like lip balm) in your bag to reapply throughout the day without any faff (and without messing up your hairline). We like Supergoop Glow Stick SPF50 (£22) or Vichy Idéal Soleil UV Stick SPF50 (£11).

The O-zone

The orbital zone is the area encircling the eyes. Eyes are the first place to show signs of ageing, but while we dutifully apply eye cream under our eyes, we're missing the crucial temple area, which is where crow's feet eventually spread. The temples are often left unprotected from the ageing sun by thinly framed sunglasses that don't offer this delicate spot adequate shade.

Solution: Give the O-zone a little TLC using cryo globes. Like dumbbells for the face, they give it a workout after a day spent squinting at screens. As well as helping with the skin's tone and texture via the stimulation of circulation, they can also help with sinus issues and headaches. And don't forget the SPF!

The J-zone

British women spend the equivalent of five years of their lives sitting at their desk/kitchen tables, and this is increasing thanks to our post-Covid extended working days. As we sit, many of us unconsciously 'rest' the sides of our face in our hands. This habit folds skin upwards, causing wrinkles around the jaw and mouth, and also redistributes the 10,000-strong army of bacteria found on your keyboard, which can clog pores and cause spots.

Solution: Use a serum that deftly tackles both blemishes and wrinkles, such as the oil-free SkinCeuticals Blemish + Age Defense

Corrective Serum (£75). Apply a double dose to the area you rest on your hand.

The sleep zone

Is one side of your face better behaved than the other? Most of us have differing hydration levels on each side of our faces, depending which side we sleep on. Your 'sleep side' is the driest, with cotton pillow cases absorbing carefully applied skincare products more than any other fabric.

Solution: Make sure you give the 'sleep side' of your face a double-duty dose of hydration come morning.

The phone zone

Our phones now live in our hands almost constantly, and with 95 per cent of people holding their phones against the left sides of their faces, this zone has become a hot spot for clogged pores. Mobile phones are covered with more bacteria than a toilet seat and that – teamed with the heat they radiate – opens pores, trapping dirt and creating an all-new blemish-prone skincare zone.

Solution: Twice a week, use Dr Dennis Gross Alpha Beta Universal Daily Peel (£18) on the area to remove debris from pores, then treat breakouts with a product containing salicylic acid. Check out our Blemish Busters section on page 24. And wipe your phone with an antibacterial wipe!

THE BEAUTY QUIZ: HOW HYDRATED IS YOUR SKIN?

Hydration is key when it comes to the look and feel of your skin, but your skin's hydration levels will fluctuate throughout the year. For example, in September, post-summer holidays and with autumn approaching, your skin might start to act out as hydration levels dip. There can be another dip come November when the heating comes on, zapping yet more moisture from the skin. This means it's a good idea to reset seasonally, check in with your skin and make sure that you're addressing its needs.

1. Pinch the skin on the back of your hand, pulling it firmly to create a tent-like shape. Hold for a few seconds, then release. Does the skin take two seconds or more to return to normal?   YES/NO

2. Over clean skin, apply a piece of transparent sticky tape to your cheek and press for three seconds. Hold it up to the light; you'll be able to see the outer layers of skin cells that have transferred on to the tape. The more dead skin cells you can see, the drier your skin is. Is the tape covered in skin cells?   YES/NO

3. Wash your face with a gentle cleanser, pat it dry and wait three hours. Now, hold a square of absorbent paper to your forehead for three seconds. Remove it; is it completely dry?   YES/NO

4. When you first step out of the shower, does the skin on your face look the freshest and plumpest it will all day?   YES/NO

5. When your skin is clean and dry, take your forefinger and place it horizontally against your cheek, then gently roll it upwards, pushing the skin. Look into a hand mirror; do you see fine horizontal lines?   YES/NO

6. After cleansing, go to bed without applying anything to your face. As soon as you wake up, touch your skin in the central zones (forehead, nose, chin and cheeks). Does it feel dry to the touch and slightly rough? Look in the mirror; does it look red, irritated or flaky?   YES/NO

7. Take a look at the skincare products you are using. If your arsenal includes soaps, toners that list alcohol as an ingredient and highly fragranced products, does your skin look pink after using them?   YES/NO

8. Hot baths or showers melt away the skin's natural protective oils. Take a long, hot bath filled with scented bubbles; does your skin feel dry and tight afterwards, as if it is being stretched?   YES/NO

9. Despite regular exfoliation and moisturising, do you still find dry skin building up in patches that feel rough and itchy (notably on knees, elbows and the backs of your legs)?   YES/NO

10. Do you find that when you look in the mirror at around 3pm, your liquid foundation has started to look uneven or patchy in places, as if it has been absorbed by your skin?   YES/NO

YOUR SKIN SCORES

If you answered 'yes' to one to two questions, your skin is:
Normal. It just needs a regular hit of daily moisture.

If you answered 'yes' to three to four questions, your skin is:
Dehydrated. This isn't a skin type, but it is a skin condition that is easily addressed by using the correct products.

If you answered 'yes' to five to six questions, your skin is:
Slightly on the dry side and in need of a thirst-quenching boost.

If you answered 'yes' to seven to eight questions, your skin is:
Dry, but this may simply be hormonal or weather-induced, so up moisture levels accordingly.

If you answered 'yes' to nine to ten questions, your skin is:
Suffering from long-term dryness. Start using products that address your skin type's specific concerns.

SKIN TYPES

Normal skin: Your skin rarely feels tight at the end of the day and you don't need to blot it to absorb excess oil. Any oiliness or dryness you do experience is rare and easily resolved. A simple switch to a moisturiser rich in ceramides and hydrating ingredients will help.

Dehydrated skin: A condition, not a skin type, so this can be fixed. Dehydrated skin can feel tight and dry in some areas while looking greasy in others. Caused by a lack of water rather than oil, make-up may become patchy throughout the day as your body compensates for the lack of moisture (which it can't self-produce) by producing more oil. Products containing glycerine and hyaluronic acid – both of which trap water – are your skin's best friends.

Slightly dry skin: This may be temporary and weather-induced. For example, cold air can reduce water content at the skin's surface, resulting in drier skin than usual. Treat it now before it becomes more serious by using slightly richer skincare products than usual.

Dry skin: Not about a lack of moisture, this is down to a lack of protective sebum (hydrating lipids) across the skin's mantle, inhibiting it from effectively protecting skin from external factors. Pores may look small and tight due to the lack of oil. Without sebum, skin appears rough and flaky, and lines are more obvious.

Uncomfortably dry skin: Ordinarily, dry skin is not a serious concern, but if it's not addressed, the deficiency in lipids and proteins can spiral, making the skin susceptible to inflammation and itchiness. Eczema – patches of skin that itch and appear inflamed, peeling and cracked – is caused by a lack of fat between the skin cells. As water evaporates, the cells shrink and cracks form between them, which are then exposed to dirt and bacteria. An emollient cream bridges the gaps so they can fill with water and swell again. Topical creams can help put it into remission. If they don't work, it's best to see your GP.

Remedying Redness

These days, many more women are suffering from skincare concerns such as rosacea and perioral dermatitis. Rosacea is a chronic skin condition thought to affect up to one in ten people. If you find that you experience symptoms of prominent redness or flushing in your skin, there's a chance it could be rosacea. Perioral dermatitis, meanwhile, is characterised as pink, scaly patches around the mouth, the cause of which is unknown; it could be genetic, hormonal or a reaction to a skincare product. Though there isn't a known cure for either condition, there is lots of research around how to reduce your symptoms and better manage them.

Rose Gallagher (@rosegallagher) is a make-up artist, content creator and rosacea expert. Here are her three skincare tips for dealing with rosacea:

1. Keep your skincare routine simple

All you need in the first instance is a cream cleanser (AM and PM), a moisturiser designed to replenish the skin barrier (AM and PM), and an SPF (AM). Look for products that are designed to repair and hydrate. You won't go far wrong with any of the French pharmacy brands; these are the brands that expert dermatologists consistently recommend to me as their go-tos.

2. Once you've found the right skincare routine, see a medical professional to identify the right active ingredients for your skin

Azelaic acid, for example, is a brilliant active ingredient for reducing the texture that can come with type 2 rosacea, but a medical professional will be best to advise on which strength you should use. Whether you visit a GP or dermatologist, or use an online skin service like the Boots Online Doctor, Klira or Skin + Me, seeking one-to-one advice is crucial as rosacea looks different for each person.

3. Keep a lifestyle diary so that you can identify patterns and manage your skin holistically

External triggers can be very powerful when it comes to exacerbating rosacea. Things like extreme weather, hot showers, eating spicy foods and drinking alcohol can all wreak havoc on your skin. By no means am I saying to avoid these things; they're all part of life. What I am saying, however, is that once you know the things that tend to disagree with your skin, you can be mindful of when you enjoy them. You could also prep ahead to minimise the impact – for example, I always moisturise before a hot shower to prevent coming out with red-hot skin.

See page 55 for tips on make-up and rosacea.

The Wind-Down

Sundays are the only time I really get to spend some time on myself. Once the kids are in bed, I retreat to the bathroom, away from the chaos of the weekend. Because of our circadian rhythms, you lose the most hydration between 9 and 11pm, so we should always aim to have our make-up off and our skincare done by then.

It can be so tricky to carve out time for yourself when you're juggling so much, but even the smallest of treats can make you feel so much better. It's all about getting it all done rather than relaxing; I need products that work fast and deliver real results. Life is too short otherwise!

I know that I won't have time in the week to do any beauty upkeep, so I do all of my essential maintenance on a Sunday. That's everything from exfoliating to tweezing my eyebrows (and random stray hairs, where do they appear from?!) and fake tanning. When it's winter I can get away with just patch-tanning, focusing only on the parts that people see, like my face and my arms.

I have different cleansers for different reasons, but on a Sunday I tend to use a balm cleanser as I have more time to play with. I also have a 'serum wardrobe'! I am a beauty editor and I am sent products to trial; you are not expected to have a wardrobe of anything, just the products that work for your skin. Still, this means that I tend to be very prescriptive in terms of what my skin needs. If I'm feeling dry, I'll use a hydrating one; if I've got some breakouts, I'll choose one with salicylic acid; or if I'm in need of some repair, I'll pick an antioxidant serum.

■ ■ ■

Now we've reached the end of the skincare chapter, hopefully you feel a little less overwhelmed and confused when it comes to the world of skincare. You are now fully armed with the knowledge you need to make the best decisions when it comes to selecting and applying your products. Go forth and glow!

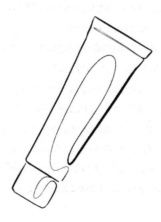

- 2 -

mastering make-up

Make-up is transformative. It's a mood booster. Of course, no one *needs* make-up, but the action of applying it and how you feel afterwards is powerful. In some cases, it can even be seen as therapeutic.

Remember those evenings spent getting ready for a big night out with your girls: music on, glasses of cheap rosé flowing, make-up spilling everywhere, sun-shimmering each other's backs and swapping application tips? How much fun were they? Then life changes, and you're more likely to be found desperately trying to scrawl on some eyeliner while the child balanced on your knee attempts to eat a blusher brush.

Typically, it's as we hit our thirties that we REALLY need our concealer to live up to expectations, our foundation to last all day and our illuminating primer (you don't use one? You will!) to, well, actually *illuminate* a tired, greige complexion.

In this chapter, I will share all the make-up tips, tricks and shortcuts I've learned over the years from my days on the backstage circuit, where make-up artists have to apply eyeliner to models as fast as a mum on the way to the school run. I'll also share the items every thirty-something needs in their make-up arsenal, and we'll look at where to really invest your time and money when it comes to make-up, so we can get your make-up bag working as efficiently as possible.

Make-up doesn't have to be complicated – especially when you're short on time.

The Psychology of Make-Up

My earliest beauty memory is watching my mum put on her make-up on a Saturday night for a 'dinner dance' in the late eighties. I kind of wish our generation went to such fancy-sounding events on a regular weekend, rather than just 'out for dinner' in jeans and a nice top. There she was, in this green taffeta puffy-shouldered ball gown, with huge earrings, hair sprayed to the max, spritzing on Anaïs Anaïs and looking into the mirror as she applied a red lipstick. Six-year-old me sat on the edge of the bath, watching. It was *so* glamorous.

Growing up around my mother's beauty salon, I saw first-hand the power that make-up has to transform a woman's confidence and project to the world the image that she wants to put across. It's the reason I became a beauty journalist in the first place.

According to a survey carried out in 2023, 92 per cent of women said their beauty routine has a significant and noticeable positive impact on their mood and well-being.[2] When women feel good about themselves, it pours into every part of their day.

The Lipstick Effect

The 'Lipstick Effect' is the theory that sales of affordable luxuries rise during economic downturns. In an economic crisis, while costly purchases such as far-flung holidays, designer bags and shoes may be avoided, customers will be more willing to buy less expensive luxury goods, such as designer lipstick, to boost their mood. The key phrase here is 'affordable luxury'.

In 2001, Leonard Lauder, chairman of Estée Lauder Companies, reported that his company saw a spike in lipstick sales after the 9/11 terrorist attacks. Meanwhile, in her 1998 book *The Overspent American*, economics and sociology professor Juliet Schor wrote that when money is tight, women will still splurge on luxury-brand lipsticks that are used in public, ready to be pulled out of one's handbag in social scenarios, such as after dinner in a restaurant, or over coffee with friends. In 2017, I wrote a blog post in a similar vein: 'For a real treat to yourself (you totally deserve it), you can't beat La Mer The Lip Balm. You'll feel incredibly chic every time you pull it out of your changing bag, even if you're sitting in the local Costa.' The idea was that new-mum life is mundane, but pulling out a luxe item in a coffee shop will give you a spike of serotonin. We also recommended teaming up and buying it as a baby shower gift, as no one gets dry lips like a woman in labour or a breastfeeding mum – although it's worth noting that at the time of the blog post, the product was *a lot* less expensive than it is now (blame inflation).

While some economists may not buy into the Lipstick Effect, data from global market tracking firm NPD Group shows that sales of lipstick and other lip make-up grew 48 per cent in the first quarter of 2022 compared to the same period in 2021.[3] That's more than twice as fast as other products in the beauty category. Now, with energy bills and mortgage payments to worry about, a less expensive yet premium-feeling purchase that gives an immediate boost is top of the agenda. Globally, beauty is expected to be characterised by 'premium-isation', with the premium beauty tier projected to grow at an annual rate of 8 per cent (compared with 5 per cent in mass-market beauty) between 2022 and 2027, as consumers trade up and increase their spending, especially on fragrance and make-up.[4]

Lipstick is transformational; it's quick, easy and needs minimal special skills, as opposed to contouring, smoky eyes or a feline flick. After Gemma and I each gave birth, our bodies didn't feel like ours, our clothes didn't fit right, but we discovered the incredible power pairing of sunglasses and a red lip. It was our saving grace during those newborn days, and we still use this trick today. A swipe of bold lipstick detracts from tired eyes, and when paired with great sunglasses – well, everyone thought that we had our sh*t together (reader, we most definitely did not have our sh*t together).

How to wear red lipstick

It might seem scary, but I promise you, lipstick is the simplest and most effective way to look instantly pulled together. Like a shot of caffeine for your face, a slick of red on the lips will make you look a thousand times more awake in just a few seconds. From a classic white T-shirt to a tailored blazer or grey sweats, it goes with everything. Plus, the stark contrast of colour also means that the whites of your eyes and teeth look much brighter. Bonus.

Our favourites all have the following things in common:

- They either come in a crayon format, a tapered lipstick bullet or as a liquid lipstick that you apply with a wand, all of which are ridiculously easy to apply.
- They are all matte. This means that, unlike their glossier counterparts, they stay put. Trust us. They don't budge.
- They don't cost the earth.

Try: Charlotte Tilbury Matte Revolution Lipstick in Red Carpet Red, £27 // Estée Lauder Color Envy Paint-On Liquid Lip in Poppy Sauvage, £27 // Smashbox Always On Matte Liquid Lipstick in Bawse, £27 // Stila Stay All Day Liquid Lipstick in Beso, £21 // Nars Powermatte Lipstick in Dragon Girl, £26 // Mac Powder Kiss Lip Colour in Ruby Boo, £24

Application tips

For a modern look, a tip I learned from make-up artists backstage at Fashion Week is to diffuse (or smudge) the edges with a cotton bud after application. This helps lipstick to stay put, and also helps it to look a bit more 'lived in' and a bit less 'done'. Then all you need to do is whack the sunglasses on and go. That's it. No one will believe that you've got ready in under thirty seconds.

★ **TIM TIP:** If that all feels a bit too high-maintenance for you, simply swipe your finger over the bullet and pat it on for more of a stain-like finish. You can build up the colour up as you get used to wearing it.

Finding Your Signature Beauty Look

I never thought that I was someone who actually *had* a signature beauty look – until I looked through our Instagram, and it quickly became pretty clear. I do. And so does Gemma. Even though there are SO MANY similarities between us (we both went to uni in Leeds, although we never met there; we gave birth in the same hospital, in the same room, in exactly the same position, three months apart, although again it was before we had even met; and we both fell pregnant with our second babies within ten days of each other, without ever having had a conversation about having second kids), we are also VERY different. Case in point: our signature beauty looks. But there's one thing we both agree on – we don't leave the house without a flick of a black eyeliner (see page 52 for our top tips on perfecting winged liner).

My signature beauty look: bronzer and a black flick
Bronzer and I have a long-standing relationship. There was a time, way back when, when I would 'triple-dip' in fake tan, using a couple of coats of wash-off over the top of a spray tan. I'll dig out pictures one day to give you a real laugh. If you went to uni in Leeds about twenty years ago, you probably did the same. Now my bronzing is slightly more subtle, but I'm still rarely seen without it.

Gemma's signature beauty look: winged liner and a red lip
Gemma is naturally fair and, despite loving a spray tan, she doesn't
have the time to dedicate to a fake-tan regime regularly, so she has
learned to embrace her natural colouring. No matter what hair colour
she has, though, she has a staple look: a bold red lip and an always
perfect winged eyeliner.

Make-up is simple. It shouldn't feel complicated or confusing. It is
better to master the basics of what suits your face and tweak it than to
buy into every single trend. By 'mastering the basics', I mean knowing
how to make yourself feel good when you look in the mirror. For us, it's
the above. For someone else, it could be a monthly facial, or a dose of
blush. For another person, they may feel entirely confident without a
scrap of make-up on their face at all. Those are the basic backbones of
beauty. Once you know what works for you, you can add the latest
trending colours – if you want.

Finding your signature beauty look will save you time and money in
the long run. Once you know what suits you and what you find easy to
wear – and, more importantly, once you master the specific make-up
techniques required – doing your make-up will take you minimal time
each morning. Over the next few pages, you'll find some of the best tips
and tricks for perfecting your own make-up techniques.

Wake-Up Make-Up: How to Look Less Tired

The most common question I get asked is, 'How do I look less tired?'
And the answer is simple: corrector and concealer. I swear – and I'm
sure all of our followers will know – that if I was stranded on a desert

island, I'd just need my Beauty Pie Superluminous Under-Eye Genius (and some SPF, obviously) and I'd be happy.

I find when I just apply mascara without using a corrector or concealer, I look more tired. This is because the eye is drawn to the area I've just emphasised, around my lashes.

What is a corrector and why do I need it as well as concealer?
A corrector uses colour theory to cancel out the tones of pigmentation so that you can conceal more easily over the top. For blue or purple undertones, use a peach or orange corrector. For brown or green undertones, try a yellow corrector.

How do I use corrector and concealer?
The trick to hiding dark circles caused by sleep deprivation is to neutralise them with a peach-hued corrector first.

Apply a thin layer of corrector in a press-push method into the darkest points of the dark circle using an angled brush (I like using the Beauty Pie Pro Angled Concealer Brush, £10 for members/£22 for non-members) to really get into that hollow corner. This allows you to use less product to counterbalance the darkness, so you can avoid that cakey look under the eyes.

Next, apply a brightening concealer under the eyes that's a shade lighter than your skin. This will brighten up the area. I like Vieve Modern Radiance Concealer (£24), which comes in twenty-plus shades. Apply small dots of concealer to the skin below the inner third of the eye, as well as the outer corner, then use an angled brush to buff it out, evening out the skin tone.

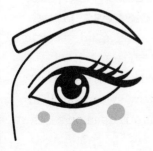
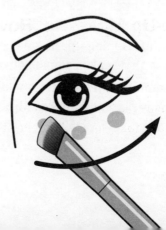

Meet Blusher: Your New Bff

Lots of people are scared of blusher. I took a while to warm up to it myself, and it wasn't until I was in my mid-thirties that I truly 'got it'. Nothing has a more instantly transformative effect than blush – it knocks off years, hides hangovers, and makes you look 'done' when you've barely had time to take off your pyjamas. Cream, powder, or stick form will all do the trick, although cream blush is my favourite.

Beauty journalist and presenter Dr Ateh Jewel launched her beauty brand Ateh Jewel Beauty in 2023, focusing entirely on blushers. Never before has a brand been able to launch into Harrods with just three shades of blush, but in 2023, Ateh made it happen.

'Beauty, to me, has always been such a beautiful safe space, as well as a prison,' she says. 'When I was fifteen, I went to a beauty counter and asked for a pink blush. I had saved up my money and was so proud and excited to use it. However, the beauty consultant said to me, "Black girls don't do blush and black girls don't do pink." She shooed me away and said I should try the back of the beauty hall, as there might be something for me there. As she spoke, she sprayed and cleaned down the counter where I had touched it, as if I was dirty. I was so devastated that she'd treated me like that. It was important [to me] that I started [my own range] with a blush that popped on all skin tones, so that everyone could enjoy it.'

Jewel explains: 'People with deeper skin tones have been naturally cautious when it comes to blushers, as most have white pigment in the base, which makes it look chalky, ashy, stuck on and doll-like. [These blushers] often don't look like part of the skin.' Jewel spent years reformulating, ripping up the rule book and starting again to create a cream blush that makes you look like you're lit up from within: 'It brings such a glow to the skin, and it doesn't settle in lines and wrinkles. It just gives your skin this amazing, bouncy, juicy, healthy glow.'

As a general rule of thumb, Jewel says, 'It's all about "undertones". I personally prefer using the colours which are cooler. People often assume because I have a black, deeper skin tone, that I automatically go for warmer tones, which just isn't true. I think everyone naturally leans towards warmer or cooler tones [depending on] which they personally prefer and love to see on their skin.'

Go for a light pink, rose or peach-toned shade if you have fair to medium skin. If you have a darker complexion, opt for tones of orange and deep berry to complement your skin. Start with a little and build up. It's easier to add more than it is to take it away.

Find the right type of blusher for you

Picking the right blush *texture* is as important as getting the shade right.

Cream blushers

These are my favourite for creating a really natural effect. They melt in, have a slight sheen, and work on almost every skin type, including dry skin. Dab a little onto your cheeks and blend with your fingers. I sometimes dab it onto my lips too.

Try: Beauty Pie Supercheek Cream Blusher, £12 members/£30 non-members.

Powder blushers

These are great for normal, oily or combination skin, but if you have dry skin, stick to cream blushers as the powdery finish just emphasises dry patches. Skip matte blusher and go for something with a glowy sheen to give you a flush that looks like it comes from the skin.

Try: MAC Powder Blusher, £26.

Gels and stains

These are longer lasting than creams and powders and are great for oilier skins, but the downside is that they aren't as mistake-proof.

Apply straight on top of foundation (not over powder) and blend quickly with warm fingertips.

Try: Glossier Cloud Paint, £20.

★ **TIM TIP:** For the most natural look, grin to identify the 'apples' of your cheeks (the parts of each cheek that fatten and rise up when you smile). Sweep your blusher brush over the top of the apple (the part that lies directly below your pupil), then blend it up and out, towards the temple. Another technique is to make the shape of an 'L' with your thumb and forefinger, then position your hand against your face so the bottom of the L (your thumb) is in line with your nose, with the tip of your thumb against your nose, and your forefinger at the side of your face towards your ear. The inner corner of your hand is where you should apply your blusher.

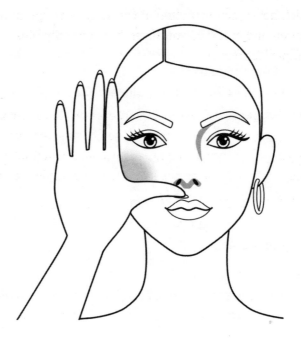

My favourite blushers: Ateh Jewel Beauty Blush of Dreams Cream Blush, £25 // Beauty Pie Supercheek Cream Blusher, £12 members/£30 non-members // Bobbi Brown Pot Rouge, £30 // Clinique Chubby Stick Cheek Balm, £25 // Westman Atelier Baby Cheeks Blush Stick, £44.

Backstage Beauty Tips for Real Life

Twice a year, packs of exhausted beauty editors roam the globe for a month during the Fashion Week circus, trekking between Paris, Milan, New York and London, dodging hot curling irons and clouds of hairspray while searching for something, anything, that will change the landscape of the beauty plains.

There are a few fundamental skills every woman should know, some of which have been forgotten in the age of Instagram make-up: how to brighten and enhance your eyes, how to apply blush, and how to conceal imperfections.

★ **TIM TIP:** Forget the carved-out smoky eyes on Instagram that use ten different shades and textures – no one has time for that. All you really need are three eyeshadows. Use the lighter shade all over the lid and the medium shade on the lid crease, then apply the darker shade with a fine brush as a liner.

How to conceal a blemish

It's important to use a shade of concealer that exactly matches your skin tone: too light and you'll only highlight the blemish; too dark and you will make it look bigger.

Use a flat brush like the Illamasqua Flat Concealer Brush (£7), to press on your concealer. Apply the formula directly on top of the spot using a dabbing motion; don't sweep it across, as this will just remove the product and aggravate the blemish.

Shimmer draws attention to the issue, so instead lightly dust a completely matte powder, such as L'Oréal Paris Infallible 24H Matte Powder (£13), over the top of the blemish to help it blend into the rest of your complexion.

How to bronze and contour

Bronzer and contour products are different things; bronzer has a warmer hue, and is used to add colour to the skin, whereas contour products are cooler toned, and are used to create shadows, sculpt and add dimension to the face with shading.

To bronze, apply your bronzer with a large fluffy brush in a 'backwards 3' shape, from temples, curling around to the centre of the cheeks, then back to the hairline and inwards to sweep along the jawbone.

To make life simpler, I use a cream bronzer stick to contour, such as Merit Bronze Balm (£32). It creates the illusion of a more sculpted face. Apply below the cheekbone and along the jawline and the temples to give depth and shadow.

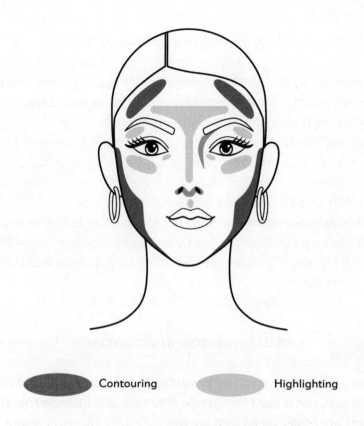

Contouring   Highlighting

How to use highlighter

Highlighter reflects light to brighten your features. Professional make-up artist Adeola Gboyega explains: 'I like to apply highlighter to the tops of the cheekbones for a subtle glow. A touch of highlighter on your cupid's bow (the area above your upper lip) can make your lips appear fuller, while a small amount down the bridge of your nose adds a natural radiance. Brighten your eyes by blending highlighter into the inner corners of the eyes; and applying a small amount beneath your eyebrows can lift your brow area.'

I always prefer a non-shimmery highlighter. Beauty Pie's Triple Luminizing Wand (member price £11/£30 non-members) is the most perfect, non-glittery, natural-looking highlighter ever. Use it on the high points of the face: the tops of the cheekbones, the temples, the bridge of the nose and under the brow bone. This will finish off your make-up with a really expert-looking pop. Apply just the tiniest bit, then buff and blend. Beautiful. It reflects the light and creates a pretty glow without any sparkle or colour.

★ **TIM TIP:** Adeola says, 'Choose champagne and pearl shades for fair skin, while gold and bronze tones suit medium to deeper skin tones.'

How to apply perfectly winged eyeliner

Rest your elbows on a flat surface and look down into a mirror. Using your ring finger, pull your eyelid taut at the outer corner, then holding your tool of choice at a forty-five-degree angle, pointing towards the outer corner of the eye, slowly glide along the lash line towards your nose until you reach the inner corner.

To wing it out, place your liner at the outer corner, drawing out and then back in the opposite direction to fill any gaps.

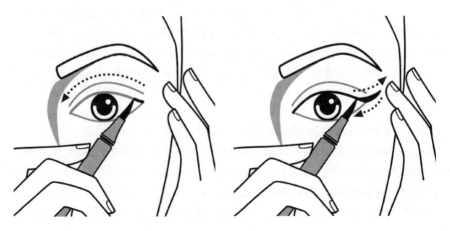

My nine-to-five job is quite fun. Among (a lot of) other things, it involves doing enough research to be able to categorically say which are the best liquid eyeliners out there. I've tried them all, from paint pots to gel wands and smoky kohls, but for inky-black goodness and real staying power, nothing beats a felt-tip applicator. I personally prefer the ease of a pen.

To pass my test, they need to: have a firm point and an even flow of ink (no one wants a rogue splat of ink just as they finish their flick); stay put (no smudging onto my eyelid, thanks); dry quickly (to withstand the smudging of tiny hands); and be great value for money (don't you hate it when a liquid liner loses its inkiness and goes grey after a couple of weeks?).

These all pass the tests above, and suit a range of budgets:

Bobbi Brown Ink Liner, £30

If you like the flick to be fairly thick but find it's too time-consuming to go back and forth over the line, this is for you. This liner stays on for hours and hours, without flaking or smudging (essential, our eyes become more hooded as we get older).

Stila Stay All Day Dual-Ended Waterproof Liner, £19

Even if you use it every day (like I do), this will be as inky black months later as it was on the day that you bought it. That's not even the best bit; it's actually two eyeliners in one, with a longer, slightly fatter applicator on one end and a smaller, finer one on the other. I draw the flick with the long side and then extend it into a lash-hugging line with the other.

L'Oréal Paris Superliner, £6.00

This is a recent discovery, but one that was well worth making. The nib is long and firm, so you can draw a fine, precise line easily, it's a proper glossy black shade, and it stays put. Like, *really* stays put. I rubbed my eyes forgetting I was wearing eyeliner, and it didn't move.

Clarins 3-Dot Liner, £22

Designed as the 'dummies guide to eyeliner', this makes wonky lines a thing of the past. Place the pen on the eyelid (precise placement depends on how winged you want your line to look), and the nib deposits three dots in a straight line. All you need to do is fill in the gaps in a dot-to-dot style for a perfectly even look.

★ **TIM TIP:** One rule we have always sworn by: don't waste money on designer mascara. High-street mascaras are brilliant. Save your money here, and invest it elsewhere in your make-up bag. Backstage secret . . . switch your black mascara for an inky navy. Blue tones brighten the whites of your eyes.

How to groom your brows

Brows are the frame to your face. You're either blessed with full, bushy brows that grow super-fast and require threading once a fortnight (Sam) or you're not (Gemma), in which case you might need to give them a little help in the right direction.

Once a month, Gemma dyes her brows at home using Eylure Dye-Brow in shade Dark Brown (£4.66). This takes fifteen minutes, and sounds so much scarier than it is. Remember to put Vaseline on the skin around your eyebrows using a cotton bud so the dye doesn't stain the skin. To fill in any gaps, Gemma uses a brow brush (see page 60) to brush the hairs upwards, then applies Beauty Pie Superbrow Luxe Precision Pencil in Hot Coffee (£9 members/£25 non-members) in light upward strokes, followed by Bobbi Brown Natural Brow Shaper in Espresso (£24) to set her brows in place.

How to cover redness

Rosé Gallagher, make-up artist and rosacea expert, has some great advice on covering redness. 'Try using a colour corrector, or CC cream, instead of a traditional foundation. CC creams are designed to neutralise areas of high colour in your skin. When it comes to covering rosacea, you might find that you have areas of completely neutral-looking skin and areas of intense flushing. A CC cream will blend naturally over both of these areas, helping to bridge the gap between them. A traditional foundation may not offer the coverage you need, and the flushing beneath may poke through like a black bra under a white T-shirt.

'Rosacea-prone skin tends to be a bit warmer to the touch, which means that make-up can melt and move a little more quickly. Take the time to check your face with every bathroom trip, and quickly top up with a touch of powder or concealer where needed. It can make a huge difference to how flawless your make-up feels all day.'

Foundation Course:
Finding the Right Foundation

The right shade of lipstick can perk up a tired face, and a cleverly chosen eyeshadow can make your eyes pop, but it's finding that shade of foundation that sits invisibly, like a second, more perfect skin, which is the real holy grail of beauty.

It's no wonder British women spend, on average, £125 and try seven different brands of foundation before finding the right one – the one that doesn't leave a tidemark around the jawline or disintegrate into patches throughout the day. It doesn't surprise me that one beauty survey found 71 per cent of women over thirty are still looking for 'the one'.[5]

But why is it so tricky? Sixty-six per cent of women have bought at least five foundations only to find they were the wrong shade, formula or texture for their skin, while 27 per cent of women are still no closer to finding the holy grail ten foundations later.

There have been many brands brought to life purely to answer this question. Il Makiage, Cosmetics à la Carte and Prescriptives (RIP) are/ were excellent online colour-matching brands, but they all rely on a great camera and good lighting. Even your local beauty counters might get it wrong, as the shade may look different inside to how it looks once you walk down the street in daylight.

I have found a great source to be the website Findation.com. If you are looking to try a new foundation then input your favourite foundations in shades that do suit you, and it will give you suggestions of what will suit you in other brands.

★ **TIM TIP:** Lancôme offer a colour-matching service at most of their counters across the country, as well as an AI-powered e-shade finder online, which can help to match you to one of their forty-five-plus shades.

Minimum Effort, Maximum Impact

We get it. Some mornings, you just can't be arsed. You feel knackered, you look knackered, your hair is dirty and there's no time to wash it. You're trying to excel in your career, maintain a social life, drink enough water, exercise, text everyone back, stay sane, survive and be happy. You don't have time for make-up. But these are the days when you always, ALWAYS bump into someone you don't want to. Like an ex-boyfriend. Or the girl who married him.

Because things like this are bound to happen on the days when you look like death, we have four ridiculously easy ways to make your usual thirty-second 'foundation and not much else' routine GLOW. Seriously. Each step takes approximately five seconds, so you're adding just twenty seconds to a 'can't-be-arsed' morning, but they will make all the difference.

Think of this approach as 'no-make-up make-up'. *Appearing* as if you're not wearing a speck of make-up isn't the same as *not* wearing a speck of make-up. The right tricks can make you look like you rolled out of bed with flawless skin, bright eyes and naturally rosy lips.

Primer

We are both obsessed with anything that makes us look glowy and wakes up our knackered, dull-looking skin. So, for the sake of a few extra seconds, get an illuminating primer into your kit! Currently on my dressing table is my Elf Cosmetics Halo Glow (£14): it's a golden, light-reflecting primer balm that rewinds my skin back to my twenties with one swipe. If redness is your problem, go for a green-tinted primer like Smashbox Photo Finish Colour Correcting Adjust Primer (£14), which colour-corrects and blurs pores and fine lines.

Blusher

We've said it before and we'll say it again: when you look exhausted, reach for the blusher. It adds a healthy shot of colour that peps up an otherwise washed-out-looking complexion.

If your skin is normal to dry, go for a cream blush without any shimmer. If your skin is oily, use powder blush and a domed, densely packed brush. Either way, look for a muted pink or berry tone that looks a little dull in the pot. Trust us, on your skin, it's the best option. And if you use a little on your lips or eyes, it brings the whole thing together in a really effortless kind of way.

Highlighter
Tired skin is dull skin, and the trick to fighting a flat complexion is always highlighter. I'm partial to a stick highlighter because, well, they're easy to use. I like to call these my 'magic wands'.

Make-up crayons
When eyeshadow sticks came along a few years ago, the make-up industry was changed for ever. They put the intensity of a cream shadow into an easy-to-use stick that was formulated to stay smudgeable for a minute, then set and last for hours without fading. Nowadays, the market is flooded with a steady stream of crayons for all make-up purpose (foundation, concealer, blusher, bronzer, contour, highlighter, eyeshadow and, of course, lip colour). Not only will they take the guesswork out of application – simply swipe and blend with your fingertips –and get you out the door ASAP, but they can also be tossed into your bag for fuss-free touch-ups throughout the day (if you have the time!). Swipe on, blend and go.

The Beauty Brush Edit

When Charlotte Tilbury first launched her make-up brand, make-up brushes were an integral part of it.

'An artist is nothing without her tools,' she told me, as we sat in her kitchen and I became one of a select few to be given a sneak peek at what would become the biggest beauty brand of the decade. With the right tools, a painter can create a work of art. The same can be said for a woman and her make-up brushes. Charlotte's brushes mimic those of a painter, with long, ergonomic handles and tapered heads. When I first tried her Eye Blender Brush, I can honestly say that my ability to create a smoky eye was transformed. It did all the hard work for me.

Spend money on your brushes: they will alter the way your make-up looks.

TIM top ten: Brushes

1. **For corrector:** Hourglass Vanish Seamless Finish Concealer Brush, £35
   A unique half-moon shape for controlled application to the contours of the face, especially under the eyes. Densely packed bristles blend seamlessly.
2. **For concealer:** Vieve Muse 119 Conceal and Prime Brush, £24
   Small, slightly pointed brush with densely packed bristles designed for precise application and blending of concealer in dark areas and crevices of the face.
3. **For foundation:** Clinique Buff Brush, £30
   Densely packed bristles and a rounded shape, perfect for applying and blending liquid or cream foundations for a seamless and flawless base.
4. **For bronzer:** Bare Minerals Supreme Finishing Brush, £29
   Soft, waved bristles gently blend powders without causing product build-up, for a naturally bronzed effect.

5. **For eyeshadow:** Charlotte Tilbury Eye Blender Brush, £25
   The long, fluffy, tapered bristles make application and blending of eyeshadows a dream.
6. **For cream blusher:** Beauty Pie Pro Angled Contour Cheek Brush, £12 members/£35 non-members
   The slanted, angled shape with dense bristles adds definition and helps sculpt the cheekbones.
7. **For powder or highlighter:** Beauty Pie Soft Highlighting Powder Brush, £10 members/£35 non-members
   Fluffy rounded bristles and a large, dome-shaped head skims the skin, ideal for applying loose or pressed powders, or blending in cream or liquid highlighters.
8. **For space-saving:** It Cosmetics Heavenly Luxe Complexion Perfection Brush, £36
   This double-ended tool has a large, fluffy, dome-shaped brush on one end that blends foundation seamlessly, and a small brush with long bristles on the other for applying brightening concealer into those nooks and crannies.
9: **For brows:** Blink Brow Bar Brow Tamer, £15
   This spoolie brush is used for brushing up brows to locate any gaps that need filling in, while also blending and grooming.
10: **For smudging kohl liner:** Elf Smudge Brush, £3
   Short and curved bristles expertly smooth shadow along the lash line for a smoky look.

A clean sweep

A few of my friends were complaining recently about how annoyingly spotty their skin is. When I asked about the last time they washed their make-up brushes, they looked at me blankly.

Cleaning your make-up brushes is one of those mundane tasks that we must all carry out. If you've spent money on your brushes, you must look after them. Each time you use your brushes, bits of make-up, oil, dirt and even bacteria can get trapped in the bristles, and remain festering in the brush after use. The next time you go to use the brush, the same thing happens, except the bacteria that has festered from the time before is now being applied to your skin. So, while it might seem basic, failure to clean your brushes can lead to clogged pores and breakouts.

Once a fortnight, give them a deep clean. There are specially formulated brush shampoos on the market (like Bobbi Brown Conditioning Brush Cleaner, £14), or a gentle children's shampoo will do the trick just fine.

1. Dampen the brush slightly with lukewarm water. Try to focus on the actual bristles, while avoiding the part of the brush where the handle meets the head, as this can loosen the glue over time.

2. Add a squirt of your brush cleanser of choice to the tip of the brush. Gently swirl the brush head around the palm of your hand to work up a lather and remove make-up from the bristles. Rinse the brush tip under running water once again.

3. Repeat step two until the water runs clear from the brush. Squeeze excess water from the brush, then use a towel to wipe your brush clean, reshaping the bristles as you go. Lay your brush flat on a small towel to dry.

4. Your brushes will need a few hours to dry after a deep cleaning, so I'd recommend washing them in the evening and leaving them to dry overnight.

★ **TIM TIP:** For a faster clean, swirl the brushes around a sieve instead of your hand. Yes, trust us. It works! In addition to a fortnightly deep clean, spritz a daily brush cleaner on your brushes after each use – we like Clinique Make-Up Brush Cleaning Spray (£15).

Faking It

Back in the olden days, also known as BC (Before Covid and Before Children), I'd get a twice-monthly spray tan on my lunch break and top up in between with a dab of fake tan here or there. In a quest to find anything that would perk me up, make me feel a bit more polished or give me a spring in my step, I've tried them all, and in the process I've created a trusty at-home fake-tan box. Seeing a flash of tanned ankle between the bottom of my jeans and my Converse really does it for me. So here's a quick rundown of my favourite fake tans, from as little as £5 a pop.

For first-timers: Isle of Paradise Self-Tanning Water in Light, £19
If you've never used fake tan before, you could still just about manage to put this on with your eyes closed and emerge with a lovely, even tan. It's *that* easy to use. Plus, it's a colour corrector, so it makes your skin look a lot more even. The formula is vegan and they're such a conscientious brand that they also offer eco-friendly refill pouches.

Sam's fave: James Read Click & Glow Drops, £19
James Read is the brainiest in the business when it comes to thinking up the quirkiest tanning offerings that you didn't even know you needed until they existed. I mix a few drops into my night cream using the palm of my hand as a mixing bowl and apply it as usual. The number of drops you add depends on the desired depth of your tan; after trial and error, I've deduced that three is my magic number.

For a buildable tan: Tan Luxe Super Glow Self-Tanning Drops, £36
Intensely hydrating with a low level of the tanning ingredient DHA, this saturates skin in moisture while gently boosting radiance. A bottle lasts a full year – oh, and it doesn't stain your pillow.

For brilliance on a budget: St Moriz Self-Tanning Mousse, £5
Loved by beauty-industry insiders, this budget buy develops into an

entirely believable tan in only a few hours, with no need to wait overnight. It also comes in a gradual lotion and a mist, but I find the mousse formula easiest to apply.

Gemma's fave: St Tropez Luxe Whipped Creme Mousse, £35
This is super-easy to apply with a mitt, so you're unlikely to miss any patches, and it smells great (*not* like biscuits!). Gemma has very pale Scottish skin, and the colour is natural-looking and believable when applied. It's packed with moisturising ingredients, hyaluronic acid and vitamin E so the tan won't fade or go patchy quickly. Wash off after eight hours, or sleep in it overnight. It doesn't transfer to sheets.

The luxe one: Sisley Self-Tanning Hydrating Facial, £110
It's pricey, but O.M.G., it's just A-MAZING. I kid you not, this is the best face tanner I have ever used. It doesn't just leave skin looking tanned, but it also makes it look flawless, healthy and young! You just need a tiny bit of the gel-cream to do your whole face, so the tube will last ages.

★ **TIM TIP:** Made a mistake? TV presenter and mum Vogue Williams understands the feeling of there never being enough time, so she created Bare by Vogue Express Tan Removal Gel (£17). 'I'm all about easy, effective products that make things simple,' she tells us. 'The fast-working gel formula works like a dream to remove stubborn tan or fix any tanning mishaps without the need to abrasively scrub the skin.' Apply liberally, leave on for five to ten minutes, then rinse off in a warm shower.

Use-By Dates

Have you had the same lip gloss for the last two years? Is your mascara going a bit crusty? How about that eye cream you use so sporadically it's lasted ages? I hate to tell you, but it's probably past its sell-by date. Take a look at the table below to see how long your beauty products will last, on average. You might be shocked.

2–3 months	1 year	2 years
mascara	lip gloss	lipstick
toner	lip balm	nail polish
active serum	moisturiser	powder
liquid eyeliner	SPF	body wash
	concealer	body lotion
	foundation	body scrub

It's actually really easy to tell how long you've got to use up a product. Look on the back of it and you should see a little symbol that looks like an open jar. The number inside that jar indicates how long a product is good for once you've started using it. For example, '12M' means twelve months.

Why does it matter? As soon as you open a product, it starts to oxidise, and it's also increasingly exposed to bacteria. Once it's past that point, it could be doing your skin more harm than good, causing irritation, inflammation, acne and worse. If you have an awful memory (don't we all?), it can be hard to keep track of all 80 bajillion bottles and tubes scattered in your bathroom. A trick we use (especially with SPF) is to write the month and year that you opened it on masking tape, then tape it on to the bottle.

The Future of the Make-Up Industry

The industry is changing but perhaps not as quickly as it could. According to make-up artist Adeola Gboyega, 'There have been significant changes in recent years to improve inclusivity and diversity in the beauty industry, but there is still work to be done. We have seen brands expand their shade ranges for foundations, concealers and other complexion products to better cater to a more diverse range of skin tones, but while this is a positive step towards inclusivity, there is always room for improvement.'

'The quality of offerings needs to be substantial; I would rather see thirty good-quality foundation offerings than fifty, and the shades need to be evenly distributed, considering undertones,' says Adeola. 'Inclusivity should extend beyond just shade ranges. It should also encompass diverse skin types, textures and skincare concerns, as well as addressing the needs of individuals with specific conditions.'

■ ■ ■

Hopefully this chapter has cleared things up a little, and saved you precious time in the mornings when it comes to applying make-up. Remember, there's absolutely no pressure, some days I am perfectly happy going make-up free, but other days we all need a little extra help – and on those days, I hope that this chapter comes in handy.

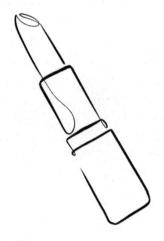

- 3 -

hair – like you just stepped out of the salon

Do you read that and hear the jingle to the Salon Selectives TV ad of the early nineties? Did you also grow up with the Timotei lady, and Jennifer Aniston telling you to buy L'Oréal's Elvive shampoo (the red one, obviously) 'because you're worth it!'? Hair language is ingrained in us and advertising tag lines for hair products are imprinted in our brains. A surprisingly large number of people will admit that hair is the first thing they notice about someone, which means your hair is communicating for you as soon as you step into a room. Within this chapter are decades' worth of time-saving tips, styling tricks, techniques and tools that will help yours speak volumes.

We are also very aware that everyone reading this book will have different hair textures and types, and it's hard to fit personal, practical advice for everyone into a single chapter with limited space and without visuals. I'm not going to pretend to be an expert in this field, but there are many experts out there, some of whom have kindly given us their words for this book. Understanding your hair is key to getting it to reflect who you are as a person, and this needn't be impossible to achieve. With a little bit of help, you can ensure that your hair tells the story you want it to, as you walk through that door.

Hair and Identity

Our hair is so intrinsically tied to our identity. When I first interviewed for my job, a rumour went around that I had the most incredible hair. I *did*. It was long, thick and voluminous. My future editor told my future colleagues that I was her 'Hair Idol'; they couldn't wait to tell me at the pub at the end of my first week's work. The pressure was then on. Every morning before work, I would prep, blow and tong my hair, making sure that it looked like I'd just stepped out of the salon. It was my confidence blanket.

These days, I'm far more low-maintenance with my hair, and we'll come on to my (irregular) wash routine soon (spoiler: it will change your life). Thanks to a smattering of greys around my hairline that are multiplying faster than Paris Fury's family (I blame my youngest child), I can no longer spread my hair colour appointments out by any longer than six weeks.

Finding the right hairdresser

One of the greatest time-saving beauty hacks for me has been to find a hair colourist and stylist whom I trust intrinsically to give me effortless colour that looks good as it fades, and cut my hair so that as it dries, it looks styled. The relationship between a woman and her hairdresser is one of the most intimate. I don't book in purely for a haircut or colour; the few hours I spend in that chair is therapy.

'Hairdressers hone their instincts over the years,' my colourist Maxine Heale at Hershesons tells me. 'We know when you need to just sit quietly, or when you want to chat through a problem. Women chat through their plans to leave their husbands; they tell us their deepest secrets. We're there to listen, unapologetically.'

Hairdressers hold a lot of power in their hands. Much has been written about this, and Charlotte Mensah, hair stylist and author of *Good Hair: The Essential Guide to Afro, Textured and Curly Hair*, agrees. 'Going to the hair salon is an intimate practice. You set aside time to focus on your hair. It can be anything from one hour to six – and this time is sacred, because you're taking time out of your usual hustle and bustle. The time set aside is special because you are choosing to create time and space to go and be wholly refreshed, both in appearance and in spirit. It's like catching up with an old friend who is also able to revitalise your whole appearance. Some of my clients have been with me for over thirty years.'

But how do you find 'The One'? My advice is to do some investigative research. If someone you know has the cut or colour you want, ask them where they go. Get busy on Instagram; it's so much easier these days to look at your local salon accounts and see which stylists they have tagged in the images you like, then follow them; you'll get a good idea of their vibe that way. Consultations are key; a good hairdresser is someone who listens to you, and takes the time to understand what you want. If you are getting a colour treatment, you must be offered a patch test beforehand to ensure that you are not allergic to the chemicals they use, and that you won't suffer any adverse reactions. No colourist worth their salt will colour your hair without requesting that you do this. A good hairdresser will also manage your expectations; if it's your first visit, chances are that they can't get your exact dream cut or colour first go, as they will be working with the remnants of previous colour processes or potentially an uneven past haircut. Give them some time to work their magic, and for the relationship to come together.

Nine Hair Hacks that Help Me Through the Week

I think people often assume that I spend hours getting ready in the morning. A fair assumption, given the nature of my job, but the reality is that I have two boys aged nine and six, and a fairly lengthy commute into town for meetings once the school run is over. This means my mornings tend to be as chaotic as they come. Over the last twenty years, I have paid attention to the dozens of hair stylists I've met, and have paired their expertise with my own personal experience to collate the best time-saving hair tips and tricks to look 'put together' in zero time. Get your hair out of a messy bun and back to its former glory. These tips, tricks and techniques will get you looking like you just stepped out of the salon – FAST. Because you're worth it . . .

1. The hair-wash routine: How to make one wash last a work week
The old 'glossy magazine' me washed her hair every other day, had a strict tonging regimen and went for regular blow-dries. The 2024 multi-hyphenated-career, self-employed, freelance, winging-it version washes it twice a week and has a tried-and-tested dry shampoo hack to make it through the work week. My best advice is to learn how your own hair behaves. No one knows better than you how long you can push a wash for, or how your hair reacts to humidity or a wind-whipping. Give this routine a try; I swore by it when I was ping-ponging between 8am meetings at the magazine and post-rush-hour nursery pick-ups, while building a fledgling business in the evenings with little to no sleep. See if it works for you.

I wash my hair on a Monday night, straighten it, then tie it into a loose bun with a silk hair tie so it doesn't kink. On Tuesday, while it's fresh, I wear it straight; on Wednesday, it has a little next-day texture, meaning waves will hold better, so I tong it; and on Thursday, I prolong wash day by spritzing it with some dry shampoo (this also gives the waves a 'cool', dishevelled texture). Fridays are for topknots before I wash it that night ahead of the weekend.

2. Use dry shampoo like an expert
Oh, dry shampoo. The saviour of tired, rushed women everywhere, because who has the time to wash their hair daily?! But there's a knack to dry shampooing right. You have to rub it vigorously with your

fingers; don't just spray it in and leave it there. Nothing else will really activate the product and help it fully absorb – and doing this boosts volume, too. This trick turns your dry shampoo into a dry blow-dry, I promise.

Try: Living Proof PHD Dry Shampoo, £19. It doesn't just soak up oil, it *removes* it.

3. Hair masks can put off a salon appointment for weeks
Nothing transforms dry, desperate-to-be-coloured hair into something far more salon-worthy than a hair mask. You might think that you don't have time, but you do. Dampen your hair under the tap in the sink, smooth on the mask from roots to tips, then twist your hair up into a bun. While the mask is doing its thing, you can get on with anything you need to be doing (placing an ASOS order or unpacking the dishwasher – your choice). Then, when you've got five minutes, jump in the shower and wash it out.

Try: Michael Van Clarke LifeSaver Leave-In Overnight Treatment, £30. We love that it comes in a huge pump bottle, rather than a tub you have to dip your hands into and then create a whole mess screwing the lid back on.

4. Give limp hair life with a texture spray
We're obsessed with texture spray. Nothing else transforms flat, lifeless hair into that off-duty-model kind of hair. I like to trust hairdresser brands when it comes to this kind of product. A good texture spray will give new life to two-day-old hair, but will also have an utterly amazing effect on freshly washed hair if yours is too soft and slippy to do anything with at first.

Try: Oribe Texture Spray, £19 // Color Wow Xtra Large Bombshell Volumizer, £24. This is formulated by Chris Appleton (he who does the hair of JLo and Kim K). It's more of a lotion that you apply to damp hair, but WOW, does it give volume.

5. All hail the mum bun . . . but do it properly

Whether you manage to wash your hair during your baby's naptime (always the aim, but more important things crop up, like, erm, Instagram scrolling) or your working week is sponsored by a can of dry shampoo and several double-shot americanos, we're all in the same boat. We find it far easier to get on with everything we have to do when our hair is out of our faces. Pull your hair into a pony and twist it until it coils over on itself before pinning.

6. Master the easy waving technique

Back in the day, I'd spend a good thirty minutes tonging my hair most mornings. These days, there's no time for that, so if I need to look pulled together for an important meeting or an interview super-quickly, I use large barrel tongs that get the job done fast. For loose, beachy waves in seconds, look for a pair without a clamp; just wrap the hair around in sections, hold for five seconds and remove the wand.

Try: Beauty Works Flat Iron Curl Bar, £55 // GHD Curve Creative Curl Wand, £150

7. Make leave-in conditioner your friend

We don't have the luxury of long, hot showers these days, so the era of a lengthy lather, rinse, repeat routine is a distant memory. Because of this, leave-in conditioner has become something of a saviour. Think of it as a moisturiser for your hair; it protects it from everything the environment will throw at it. It also means that if you have to run out of the door sans blow-dry, your hair won't frizz up. The professionals call this air-drying. See, you're totally on trend.

8. Dry your hair faster

If you do have time to blow-dry your hair, congrats. For those of us who don't, a good blow-dry spray could be what you've been searching for. Spritz throughout damp hair, then blow-dry. It will cut drying time by 30 per cent, thanks to a crystal-clear polymer that 'squeezes out' excess water so hair can dry faster. However much time you have in the morning, this means that you can hit snooze once more. And who wouldn't want that?

Try: Color Wow Speed Dry Spray, £16

9. Find a great colourist

One of the most game-changing things for me has been to find a great hair colourist, and keep them. I see Maxine Heale at Hershesons for my colour. And because I always get DMs asking what I have done, I asked her specifically for you.

She told me: 'To achieve your colour, we start by applying an all-over base colour [which Maxine calls the 'tint']. This generally covers any grey hairs and makes it look rich and glossy [recreating a similar base shade to my natural hair colour as a child]. Next, we irregularly lighten pieces using a balayage style technique, either freehand or in foils if we want to go lighter in the summer. The final stage is the toner at the basin [this is where the magic happens]'. Maxine describes the toning shade as like shading in a picture. It adds depth and movement. We generally go for a cooler, glossier tone – toffee, milk chocolate, salted caramel shades – for the most expensive looking brunette.

Over the past eight years, we've never drastically changed my colour; we stick to subtle colour tweaks, expertly blended so it's hard to put your finger on whether we've gone a bit darker or a bit lighter, dialling the light pieces up in the summer and down in the winter, when we add a chocolatey gloss. It's a low-maintenance colour technique, and it's all in the way that it grows out. Even though I'm brunette, Maxine told me to use a purple hair mask for blond hair to stop any of the lighter bits from going brassy or orange.

★ **TIM TIP:** When it comes to concealing greys, I swear by L'Oréal Paris Magic Retouch Temporary Instant Root Concealer Spray (£4). Just don't apply it while wearing a white T-shirt.

Power Up: The Hair-Tool Edit

How did you style your hair this morning? Did your arms struggle under the weight of a huge chunk of blow-drying apparatus? Did your right arm go tingly from being contorted into awkward positions? Did it take you twenty-seven minutes that you didn't really have? And did your hair still not look quite right? The right hair tool is worth its weight in gold, but finding it is tricky territory to navigate. Hair tools can promise – and cost – so much, and often they simply don't deliver. Here are nine that are tried, tested and have the TIM seal of approval, whatever style you're going for.

1. The hair wand: Beauty Works Flat Iron Curl Bar, £55
Whenever you see either of us with our hair wavy, it's highly likely that we've used this. Rather than a traditional cylinder shape, this wand is more flattened, as if someone has squashed your tongs, but its shape gives those really tousled, beachy waves that we both prefer. We like a wand over a more traditional tong, because it doesn't come with a clamp; simply wind your hair around it, hold for ten seconds, then let it drop off the wand into your hand. This wand comes in two sizes; I use the chunkier, shorter size for my mid-length hair, and Gemma uses the longer, narrower size for her very long hair.

2. The multi-styler: Shark Speed Style 5-in-1, £250
Hot on the heels of Dyson, the Shark Speed Style offers a great alternative for the price. The hairdryer itself is super-light and super-fast (similar in weight to the Hershesons dryer below), with five extra attachments so you can tailor it to your style. Compared to the Dyson, it's fair to say you get what you pay for; the waving barrel is shorter here, meaning that it's not so great for long hair, but those with shorter lengths will be fine. It's also less ergonomic, as you have to twist the barrel with your other hand to wave the hair – but it's about half the price.

3. The crimper: Mermade 3 Barrel Hair Curler, £20

Yes, you read that right. Crimping is coming back into fashion – but not as we know it. Forget the eighties; modern-day crimpers have wider plates, meaning you get more of a mermaid finish, like Sydney Sweeney in *White Lotus*. Simply take large sections of hair, and clamp down from root to tip.

4. The straightener: GHD Max, £165

The OG. You just know with GHD that you're getting quality. We swear by this straightener, with the extra-large plates (70 per cent larger than the average) giving you sleek, smooth hair in double-quick time. They heat up within thirty seconds and automatically switch off after thirty minutes of non-use.

5. The hairdryer under £50: Babyliss Hydra-Fusion Air Dryer, £45

It might not have all the bells and whistles of the fancier models, but it does what it says on the tin. Gemma has oodles of hair and finds that this dries it in under ten minutes.

6. The pro hairdryer: Hershesons Great Hairdryer, £295

Lighter, faster and better than any other hairdryer we've ever used. It weighs the same as a can of Coke and dries hair 30 per cent faster than anything else, making it the perfect travel companion. It comes complete with three different drying attachments – a narrow nozzle, a wide nozzle and a diffuser – so it works whether your hair is long, short, fine, thick or curly. Looks pretty chic, too.

7. The hair tong: Babyliss Titanium Brilliance Hair Curler, £28

A lot of people prefer using a tong with a clamp rather than a wand, which traps the hair under the lever for more of a controlled curl. If this is you, these tongs are a brilliant price and give a really cool-looking curl. Section hair and wrap each section the full way down the barrel for a glamorous-looking wave, or leave the very ends of your hair out of the clamp rather than curling them for more of a relaxed, undone look.

8. The ultimate tool: Dyson Airwrap Complete Multi-Styler, £480
I think we can all safely say that if you're looking for the best multi-styler around, this is the one. It dries, it waves, it curls, it delivers a big bouncy blow-dry; it even smooths and sleekens hair now, thanks to the new attachment. A hefty investment, but when you consider it does EVERYTHING, turning you into a hairstylist in the comfort of your own home – and without an ounce of arm ache – it can be justified.

9. Heatless curlers
In 2023, TikTok finally gave us something that was really and genuinely helpful: heat-free curlers. You don't need to splash out on a set, though, your dressing-gown cord will do perfectly when it comes to creating these viral, foolproof waves . . .

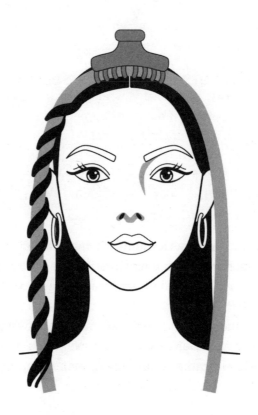

Step 1: Begin with damp hair. You could run some oil through the ends if your hair needs it. Part your hair in the middle.

Step 2: Put the belt or cord on your head, with the sides draping down evenly. Using a claw clip, secure the belt at the top of your head, level with the tops of your ears.

Step 3: Start twisting the hair around the cord, working from the front backwards, picking up more hair as you go.

Step 4: Leave overnight.

Step 5: Remove by taking off the clip and unravelling the hair. Shake out. Use a little serum or hair oil to tame the curls.

Our Best-Kept Hair Secret

We spend fortunes on skincare, but just a few centimetres north of our faces lies what is often one of the most neglected areas of our bodies. The skin on your scalp is really just an extension of that on your face, yet it rarely gets a look-in when it comes to treatments. Oil, daily grime and product residue (especially dry shampoo) can really bed in on the scalp, throwing the skin's microbiome off-balance and leading to a host of problems, from excessive dryness and flaking to oiliness and stunted growth. But treat your scalp well, and it will be able to produce strong, healthy, shiny hair.

It might not sound sexy, but using a scalp scrub every couple of weeks, or switching out our regular shampoo once a week and washing with an exfoliating formula, is our biggest hair secret. And we promise: if you do this too, you will see a real difference.

In the summer, you'll notice the benefit even more, as a scalp scrub can unclog blocked hair follicles filled with sweat and SPF that weigh your hair down.

Some scrubs use grainy exfoliators like salt or sugar, while others dissolve gunk using chemical exfoliants like salicylic acid. A scrub will last you ages, too, as you only use it a couple of times a month. Here are some of our tried-and-tested firm favourites.

Michael Van Clarke Exfoliating Scalp Shampoo, £25
This is pretty much the entire reason that Gemma's hair has reached the length it has. Designed for weekly use, the fruit acids in this shampoo cleanse the scalp, lifting away product build-up, leaving both hair and scalp feeling super-clean and fresh but never stripped. Added bonus cashmere proteins penetrate deep into the hair shaft, meaning that hair grows stronger and thicker.

Kerastase Chronologiste Pre-Cleanse Hair Scrub, £25
Apply this black gel-like formula to the scalp, massage it in and leave it to do its job for five minutes before hopping in the shower and shampooing as usual. This one leaves your hair light as air, and as swishy and glossy as if you've just had a salon blow-dry. Ideal if you live in a city, as it dissolves 96 per cent more pollutants that cling to hair than a regular shampoo does.

Drunk Elephant TLC Happi Scalp Scrub, £30
This is the one that first got us hooked all those years ago. The nozzle makes applying direct to the scalp in sections a doddle; just massage in, wait five minutes, then rinse your hair as usual. The AHA/BHA acid blend quickly breaks down and dissolves dead skin cells and product build-up, while biodegradable cellulose beads help exfoliate and detoxify the scalp. You'll see results immediately after the first use. Smells like cherry Bakewell tart.

Afro Hair

For anyone with curly hair who hasn't been lucky enough to find their hairdressing soulmate, hair stylist Charlotte Mensah's book *Good Hair: The Essential Guide to Afro, Textured and Curly Hair* is a manual for understanding afro curly textures, and shows readers how to celebrate and love their curls. Mensah's book offers a very affordable hands-on hair workshop on how to care for your hair, maintain it and keep it healthy.

'We live in increasingly diverse societies across the UK, and for me, what diversity and inclusion truly represent are the options that are available to people,' says Mensah. 'Let's take a young Black woman, living in Wales; irrespective of what the general demographic of the area is, a truly diverse society would cater for her haircare needs. It doesn't have to be another Black person, but it must be someone who has specialist knowledge on afro hair. The inclusion of afro hair on the national curriculum that apprentices must go through would create a breed of stylists ready to deal with all kinds of hair wherever you are in the country.'

It's clear from looking at the offerings in most high-street hair salons that as a society we can always be doing more to be inclusive.

Charlotte's at-home advice for afro hair

Massage the scalp
Take a few minutes each day to massage your scalp with Charlotte Mensah Manketti Hair Oil (100ml £52). This simple practice prompts the secretion of sebaceous oils and stimulates blood circulation.

Wash your hair once a week
Oils are your friend. The Charlotte Mensah Manketti Oil Shampoo (£26)

nourishes dry and unmanageable strands and keeps hair hydrated and soft. Follow by using Manketti Oil Conditioner (£26), which is a rich, creamy formula that replenishes a lot of moisture, whilst protecting the hair.

Use product cocktailing to customise your haircare regime
Product cocktailing is simply mixing two or three products together to meet your specific styling needs. My favourite cocktails are curl cream plus Manketti Oil Pomade, a tiny amount of styling gel and some Manketti Oil – this allows for a supreme hold without leaving your hair dry and crunchy.

Afro hair is fragile and needs to be treated with the gentlest of care in order for it to flourish
Paddle brushes, wide-tooth combs and natural ingredients are the best tools and products for natural hair. Low manipulation and protective styles help to retain length, because constant grooming can be too much for some hair types, especially 4C (the tightest curl type in the curl pattern).

The three biggest misconceptions about afro hair

Natural hair doesn't grow
Afro hair in its natural state tends to shrink up, preventing you from seeing its real length.

You can grow your hair if it's destined to grow. Hair grows on average half an inch per month, so your hair *is* growing, but you may not be retaining the length due to chemical abuse, excess heat styling and a general lack of proper care.

Split ends can be repaired with products
Once the hair has split, it cannot be repaired. There are products that

advertise repair and temporary mends, but the only way to get rid of split ends is to trim them every six to eight weeks.

Silk scarves and silk pillowcases aren't necessary
Cotton scarves and pillowcases can cause friction on already naturally porous textured hair. Wrapping your hair in a silk scarf will help to promote healthier, shinier hair, and help to keep your hair soft, moisturised and free of tangles.

You Are W-Hair You Live

Did you know that where you live can affect the condition of your hair? Sixty-five per cent of UK women spend at least £100 on hair products per year,[6] but you may as well throw that in the sea if you aren't targeting the real cause of your hair complaints. Some of your biggest hair problems can be attributed to your postcode. From the humidity-destroying cool air in the north-west of the UK to the colour-fading UV hotspots of the south-east, where we live can have a real impact on the state of our hair, without most of us even realising it.

Dull hair caused by hard water
Found in, for example, Brighton, Bristol, Hull, Lincoln, London, Norwich, Southampton
As anyone from the hard-water areas of Greater London and the south-east who has showered in the soft water of Glasgow or Belfast knows, it's like hair awakens from the dead to become a shiny, perky, hair-ad version of its former self, all thanks to the fresh water pumped from the lochs and lakes nearby. 'Hard water' occurs when water passes through rocks as it is pumped from underground, absorbing minerals such as calcium and copper, which then deposit on to hair fibres when

showering. Minerals fracture and erode the lipids and proteins needed for healthy-looking hair. Fractured surfaces don't reflect light very well, so colour looks dull and matte.

Treat it: Antioxidant technology uses 'mineral magnets' to target, capture and deactivate copper. Try Hello Klean's Hard Water Shampoo (£20), or Kérastase Première Decalcifying Repairing Shampoo (£32) which decalcifies hair, repairing from within.

Grey hair caused by pollution

Found in, for example, Greater London, Greater Manchester, Nottingham, Swansea, Tyneside, West Midlands

A vein of pollution courses its way from London up the M1, wrapping around Britain's over-populated cities. When toxic pollution builds up on hair, it damages the surface proteins, creating free radicals that fragment the structure of hair cells. Some studies show that this causes premature grey hairs.

Treat it: There is no cure for grey hair (and genetics play a big part!), but by ensuring pollution doesn't build up, you can stop accelerated ageing. Cleanse grime from the scalp with an antibacterial shampoo like Vichy Purifying Shampoo (£13), or try a scalp scrub (see page 77).

Dry hair caused by high wind speeds

Found in, for example, Inverness, north Wales, Pembrokeshire, western Scotland

Western Scotland is one of the windiest parts of the UK; high pressure over Scandinavia brings strong, westerly winds and, with them, sea air. Salty air literally sucks the hydration out of hair; that's why salt sprays are used for a matte finish in styling.

Treat it: Pureology Hydrate Hydra Whip Masque (£21) sells best on the Welsh coast, reflecting the drying nature of a sea breeze. By strengthening hair with mask usage, hydration levels are better locked in, making it harder for moisture to escape.

Lather, Rinse, Repeat: Reading the Label

Hair product labels have a lot to answer for. All that jargon can be SO confusing. If you've ever read the back of your shampoo bottle while waiting for your conditioner to do its thing, you'll get it. What does it all mean? Here's a quick breakdown.

Sulphates
Sulphates are the main cleansing ingredient in a shampoo, and they are what create the lather. Sensitive scalps may find these irritating. There are some excellent sulphate-free brands, like Pureology.

Silicones
These seal the hairs' cuticles, making your locks super-shiny. They're found in a lot of supermarket-brand hair products. They build up on hair over time, which isn't necessarily bad, but those with fine hair should avoid, as they weigh down the hair.

Parabens
This group of chemicals is used to prevent harmful bacteria from forming, and keep products 'fresh' for longer. Their use is controversial and they are often demonised, although they're safe in small quantities.

Proteins
Proteins, such as soy amino acids, are added to conditioners to strengthen hair. They are good for all hair types.

■ ■ ■

As we've discussed, everyone's hair is different. Is your hair dry, greasy or a little bit of both? Frizzy or over-processed? Damaged? Weak? Coarse and curly, or fine and poker-straight? There's no 'one size fits all' in the world of haircare. As with everything in this book, the advice we've shared in this chapter has been tailored to fit into the lives of people who don't have much time to spare. The best course of action when it comes to hair is to try to understand yours a little better, and weave in the advice in this book where it works for you.

- 4 -

beauty as therapy

In this chapter, we're going to change the pace a little. You can't have missed the headlines about the growth of the health and wellness industry over the last decade; globally, it was valued at over $5 billion in 2022. While I personally don't buy into the mass commercialisation of wellness, it's so important to look at the 'good' within the beauty sphere as an antidote to the current pandemic of overwhelm affecting women.

About six years ago, I left my dream job as the beauty director of the UK's most-read women's weekly magazine. I had worked at the magazine for almost eight years, and in the industry for thirteen years. It was a job that defined me (or so I thought), but even though my working life revolved around giving beauty and lifestyle advice to hundreds of thousands of women a week, I was a husk of my stressed-out self, with the breakouts and bad sleep to prove it. On the outside, my life was glossy, but internally, the stress was eating me up.

Burnout isn't just everyday stress, nor is it depression or anxiety. Burnout is all-consuming; it's sacrificing tiny, seemingly insignificant pieces of yourself, your sleep and your time, until it feels as if you're drowning.

Back in 2019, the World Health Organization recognised burnout syndrome as a legitimate medical concern, adding it to the International Classification of Diseases list for 2020. Fast-forward to 2021, and as we stepped out of a global pandemic and found ourselves catapulted straight back into the fast-paced lives we'd been forced to put on pause, the feeling of being frazzled reached new heights.

Searches for 'burnout symptoms' in the UK rose from 1,000 in August 2016 to 3,600 in August 2020, and 12,100 in August 2021. This represents a 260 per cent increase from 2016 to 2020, and a further 260 per cent increase between 2020 and 2021.[7] Another year on, in August 2022, 88 per cent of UK employees said they had experienced at least some level of burnout over the last two years.[8]

Is Burnout the New Pandemic?

Three years on from the pandemic, there are few signs burnout is abating. While remote and hybrid working are said to have afforded employees greater work–life balance, flexibility can also come at a price. In this new world, we are accessible wherever we are, round the clock. Workdays have extended, as we fit work around our family during 'flexi' hours. Add to this the post-pandemic stresses of inflation, the housing crisis and the risk of unemployment, and it's little wonder that symptoms of burnout are brewing.

I loved and lived my job. A promotion coincided with my return from maternity leave, and I was determined that motherhood would not become the full stop at the end of my CV. Four days a week, I'd flit between meetings with beauty brand CEOs, conceptualising the weekly beauty pages, shooting, writing and travelling internationally for work, before downing tools (and donning trainers) at 4.59pm to *run* for the train and collect my two-year-old son from nursery. I'd fall through the nursery door at 6.01pm, his face crumpling as they vacuumed up around him. My Fridays, which were supposed to be about spending time with him, were spent completing work I hadn't managed to squeeze into the other four days, and my evenings were spent building a nugget of an idea – This is Mothership – into the early hours.

Cumulative work stress is a big contributor towards burnout, but the first signs often emerge at home. I may have looked like I was acing it on the job front, but at home we ate cereal for dinner at least once a week because I'd forgotten to do the online shop. I skipped pages of my son's bedtime story in order to return to my emails quicker, and my to-do list was out of control. It felt like I'd been blindfolded after ten espressos and put into a tumble dryer. I was exhausted yet wired; I was bad tempered, anxious and always in a rush. My thoughts were scattered around my head like a dropped deck of playing cards, and I couldn't sleep. Despite my bone-dead exhaustion, I would wake at 2am thinking about work dilemmas and email myself notes in case I forgot my ideas by morning. But it wasn't until I had my adrenals tested for a feature I was working on that I realised something was very wrong.

Holistic GP and hormone specialist Dr Sohère Roked tested my hormone levels via four saliva swabs taken at intervals during a regular working day. She called me after hours with the results. It sounded serious.

'Your cortisol levels are abnormally high all day, spiking when you wake up and again at around 4pm. If your cortisol and adrenaline levels remain this high, you will burn out within two years,' she told me.

Roked sees many women in her clinic suffering from what's being described as adrenal fatigue or 'city syndrome': a stress-induced state where your adrenal glands (the two walnut-sized ones sitting atop your kidneys) are on constant high alert. When called upon to exert the fight-or-flight response over and over, these adrenal glands simply accommodate by switching to low battery mode; until they have a chance to fully recover.

'Each of us has a different engine when it comes to burnout, and each of us will present differently when that engine starts to slow down and malfunction because it can no longer keep itself running,' explains Joanna Ellner, acupuncturist and founder of skincare brand REOME.

'This is when you "burn out". As well as the usual symptoms of burnout (moodiness, exhaustion, over-caffeinating), there are less obvious ones: headaches, muscle pain, indigestion, trouble conceiving, and allergy flare-ups.'

But, as Charlotte Silver, life coach and mentor (and my sister-in-law) explains, 'Generically speaking, everyone – no matter their background, race, religion, social status or finances – is able to make some minor well-being changes in their lives. And the smallest of changes can be life-changing to those who are living in a state of constant bubbling under the surface, like a fuse ready to blow.'

Charlotte suggests that when you find yourself in a classic 'about to blow' scenario, take a beat and think about 'who' you are being in that moment. 'Are you who you want to be when you shout at your kids because *you* need peace after a hectic day? Are you who you want to be when you put your mum on speakerphone and ignore her with an intermittent "yeah" because *you've* had a bad day? Are you who you want to be when you bring low energy into a room with your partner because *you're* living out of alignment, but you can't bring yourself to talk? All of these people are getting the worst version of you.'

Time for you

I have an issue with the wellness industry and the way that it's commercialised our need to slow down. Even finding calm costs you these days. Giselle La Pompe-Moore, author of *Take It In*, speaker and slow-living advocate, agrees. 'If well-being practices are supposed to help us to be well, then they really shouldn't be an extra source of stress and expense for us,' she says. 'Quiet joys are always available when we slow down for long enough to notice them. It might be the voice note from your friend that made your ribs ache from laughing so much. It could be a tuna sandwich that took your breath away. It might be taking your bra off after a long day or the sunset from your garden.

This is a precious reminder that the beauty of life often exists in the small moments.'

According to a 2023 study conducted by Sanctuary Spa, women get only seventeen minutes of 'me time' a day. To some, even that may sound like a lot. To others, it's laughable. It's less time than an episode of *Friends*. Is it any wonder we're turning into an army of zombies?

'We swallow life; we say we're fine when in fact we aren't,' explains facialist Anastasia Achilleos, whose words will ring true for many. 'We're so unconnected to ourselves that we don't even know it.'

Following the pandemic, during which we were forced to forgo the spas and salons as a place to relax, a new breed of beauty products emerged that promised to do more, healing us from within our own bathroom walls.

Beware of marketing hype. 'Although largely well-intentioned, the term "self-care" has unfortunately been overly commodified and commercialised since its inception around ten years ago and, as such, has lost much of its core meaning,' Joanna Ellner points out. '"Self-care" is now synonymous with cheap, throwaway beauty culture: bath bombs, panda eye masks, hashtags and two-for-one deals, most of which are highly wasteful. Beyond that, it's also infused with notions of being self-indulgent, superfluous and a bit silly. I absolutely refute that. If anyone could benefit from "self-care", it's the over-achieving, thirty-something, working mother.'

In traditional Chinese medicine, 'self-care' is not seen as remotely indulgent or lazy. '*Yang-sheng*, or "self-cultivation", is seen as an indispensable daily practice that enhances our longevity,' says Ellner. She describes it as 'any daily practice that busies the hands and quiets the mind, traditionally taking the form of slow-moving practices such as Tai Chi, gardening or painting'. However, Ellner strongly believes that Western notions of 'self-care', including bathing, skin practices and rituals, and even applying make-up can be considered as forms of *yang-sheng*. 'And,' she notes, 'they're some of the few remaining activities available to us that remove the need for a digital screen. And that's something worth protecting.'

Giselle La Pompe-Moore points out that it's so easy to feel overwhelmed, distracted and disconnected when it feels like there's so little time to just *be* with ourselves. But that's exactly where the medicine is. She is adamant we can all do it, and uses meditation as an example: 'Throw out the rule book.' You can't get meditation wrong; you're going to think a whole lot of thoughts as soon as you

---

Tips from life coach and mentor Charlotte Silver to help keep your mind calm in those moments where you feel like you could explode

Stay present
We all hate being told to 'slow down'. It's easier said than done when we have busy lives and families to care for. 'The past is history; it's gone. The future is unknown. Bring yourself into the present moment because that's all we have,' says Silver. 'We can't control our circumstances and we can't control our thoughts. What we *can* control is our response in the present moment, to both of these things, which impacts how we act, feel and, most importantly, who we're *being*.'

Be curious
We don't all come from the same perspective; we don't all see life through the same lens. No one is against you, although it may seem like it at times. 'Become curious about where the other person's viewpoint is coming from,' says Silver. 'Understand your own viewpoint and why you see things the way that you do. How could you see and do things differently? Navigate others with the same curiosity. It's okay to not always agree.'

do it, and that is perfectly okay. You don't have to meditate for twenty minutes. If your schedule only allows for two minutes, then set a timer, breathe in and repeat the word "in" in your mind, then breathe out and repeat the word "out"; keep doing this over and over until the time runs out. You can do it in your pyjamas in bed. You don't need a twenty-five-step morning routine. If your well-being practices only last as long as the ad breaks between your favourite shows, then it's enough.'

My message is: take some time out for yourself, even to lock yourself in the bathroom. Rather than simply adopting a 'slap and go' approach, look for specific formulas and rituals that can have a huge impact when it comes to balancing, calming and restoring the body, skin and mind.

TIM Top 10: From Burnout to Beauty Breakthrough, Products that Work

REOME Active Recovery Broth, £75
A unique healing serum backed by traditional Chinese medicine, this balances yin and yang to soothe tired, stressed skin, restoring it to health. Expect calm, nourished, hyper-hydrated, radiant, plump skin within weeks. Press into the skin, concentrating on pressure points.

Aveda Chakra 1 Balancing Body Mist Grounded, £30
This was the scent of the offices at *Stylist*, a busy, bustling, weekly magazine with tight deadlines. At least daily, when dealing with a particularly stressful scenario, someone would shout, 'Get out the Chakra spray!', and we'd all spritz with wild abandon. The blend of pure essential oils is linked to the root chakra in Ayurveda, an Indian form of healing medicine that brings good energy.

Mio Liquid Yoga, £27
Another product I relied on heavily when working in a high-pressure environment, this was created to inspire the same sense of tranquillity

found post-yoga, with scents of lavender and eucalyptus to calm and soothe. Add a capful to running water and breathe.

Beauty Pie Goodie Two Chews Zen O'Clock Calming Gummies, £30:
Vegan, chewable daily supplements blended with chamomile, L-theanine and vitamin B6. These help support the nervous system, and reduce tiredness and fatigue. Take two a day.

NEOM SOS Calming Pen, £20
Cramped commute? Long meeting? Looming deadline? Try an on-the-go scent solution. The ritual of rolling this on to wrists is as good a calming factor as the soothing scent.

Spacemasks, £17
A self-heating eye mask that releases tension around your eyes and temples, and really does help you relax. Bonus points; you can't look at your phone/reply to emails/do housework while wearing it – it's forced relaxation. Zone out.

Bed of Nails Accupressure Mat, £70
Eastern wisdom meets Scandinavian modernity in this acupressure mat, which has more than 8,800 non-toxic plastic spikes. The spikes work in a similar way to acupuncture needles, helping release endorphins (the body's own 'happiness' drug) and oxytocin, to help you stay calm and relaxed. From soothing sleeplessness and easing stress to alleviating aches and pains, the spikes help the body rid itself of toxins, increase blood flow and help you get a heavenly night's sleep.

@fireflyformula Gua Sha and Face Yoga
If you find that you hold a lot of tension in your jaw, grind your teeth at night or suffer from tension headaches, you might want to try gua sha. Carelle Rose (@fireflyformula) offers a monthly online tutorial for £30 a month, but her Instagram page is packed with easy tutorials you can do at home, and her before-and-after images of facial structures are mind-blowing.

Jo Malone London Pomegranate Noir Candle, from £28
This is the ultimate candle to cosy up with. Sometimes just the act of lighting a candle and watching the flame flicker is enough to distract you from what's whirring around your brain. To me, lighting a candle after I close my laptop at the end of the day is a signal: 'the evening is now yours'. The 'me time' can begin. When we gaze at a flickering flame, the brain begins to shift out of the beta brainwave state, which is associated with thinking and alertness, and into the alpha brainwave state, which corresponds to a relaxed and creative state of mind.

Fraîcheur Ice Globes, £30
Twitchy eyes are often a sign of being over-screened and over-stressed. The relief that comes from rolling a set of these over your eyes, cold from the fridge, is incomparable. Not only do they de-puff (soothing after a night of broken sleep or a crying session), but they also help boost circulation, giving skin a glow.

Shower or Bath?

The world falls into two camps; those who prefer a shower and those who love a bath. Personally, I cannot tell you the last time I had a bath. Taking a shower means I'm not inclined to check my phone, which is definitely a good thing, as I can fall easily into an Instagram hole. Yet there are those who swear that a bath is the only way they can relax and switch off, and, more importantly, who believe a bath will soothe any manner of illnesses. Whatever camp you fall into, enjoy it, because truthfully, the only time we're *really* alone – away from people and technology – is in the bathroom.

The bath lovers

Many believe that a bathtub is both is a self-help haven and a wellness cauldron. Having trouble sleeping? Take a bath. In order to prepare for sleep, the body needs to cool down by half a degree; the sudden drop in body temperature when hoisting yourself out of the tub accelerates this cooling. Sore back? Soaking for twenty minutes in water at forty degrees (the optimum temperature to expel toxins) can increase lymph flow, causing blood to rush to the skin's surface, relaxing muscles. For period pains, adding a dash of clary sage to your bathwater (try The White Company Sleep Relax Bath Oil, £35) helps to dilate the constricted blood vessels that cause cramps. Got a cold? Sprinkle in a little of Goop's Nurse! Under The Weather Bath Soak (£24), an antibacterial blend of manuka and eucalyptus.

The power showerers

At work, we try too hard. Science states that you're more likely to have an epiphany when doing something mindless, as these mundane tasks free up your subconscious to work on something else. The ideas formed in the shower differ to those you come up with in the office because your prefrontal cortex (the brain's command centre) is relaxed.

But are you an 'everything shower' kind of person, lathering up for a full-body scrub, double-cleanse, hair wash *and* mask, or do you just take a quick, perfunctory cleanse most mornings? Seventy-five per cent of women over thirty say they get less than an hour of 'me time' per day, and of these, thirty per cent say it's less than half an hour.[9] We are a generation of busy, multi-tasking, ball-juggling women. As a result, beauty brands have answered our calls for products that work overtime, just like we do.

Products to power up your shower and reclaim vital minutes

- **St Tropez In-Shower Tanning Lotion, £28**
  The water-accelerated DHA tanning agent in this lotion gives you a Giselle-worthy tan – with no stained sheets.
- **The Sanctuary Wet Skin Moisture Miracle, £8**
  This is a game-changer for the time-poor. It's a hydrating body lotion designed to be applied to wet skin and then towelled off, leaving behind a sheath of moisture. The developers describe the technology as 'like buttering warm toast rather than bread'. Makes perfect sense.
- **Living Proof Perfect Hair Day In-Shower Styler, £13**
  Apply in the shower, then rinse off and let hair air-dry. This is packed with patented thickening molecules and intense conditioners for relaxed, glossy hair.

Help at Home

While we know that glossy hair does not a CEO make, the truth is that whether we like it or not, appearances *do* matter in the modern world. But in this 'work from home' era, where we're actually working longer hours than ever before, it's hard to find time for a cup of tea, let alone anything more. If you, like me, are covering your greys with copious spritzes of root touch-up spray, walking around on feet that haven't seen a pedicure station in months, or sighing daily at your chipped nails, you will know precisely how difficult it is to eke out an hour or two in which to make yourself look presentable, while finding three hours to get your highlights done seems to be verging on indulgence.

Luckily, there are evolving beauty services emerging that make regular grooming an achievable reality for busy women. Ruuby, the at-home beauty service, is leading the way, 'Deliveroo-ing' qualified professionals to your door, be it for a 6am blow-dry, a 9pm gel mani, a much-needed osteopathy treatment, some reflexology, or a quiet sneaky pedicure while you're in a Zoom meeting. Whether you're a working woman or a new mum with only a lunchtime nap to spare, there *are* now enough hours in the day.

My hope is that this chapter, while not a traditional beauty guide, has armed you with some tools that will help you to find a sort of balance amid the chaos. My personal advice to anyone feeling a sense of overwhelm is that rather than leaning in, it's often more beneficial to lean *out*. Reframing 'how' and 'why' I work was the key to my recovery from burnout. As an ex-editor told me, replying to emails outside of work hours doesn't make you look diligent, it suggests that you can't handle your workload. These days, my laptop stays in my study, no longer joining my husband and me on the sofa in the evenings, and I grab 'micro moments' of 'me' time whenever I can, even if that's something as simple as getting to the school gate five minutes early, to have a quick moment of calm before the madness commences.

■　■　■

I hope this beauty section has been insightful and useful, helping you to feel confident in a world that sometimes seems determined to send our heads spinning with complicated jargon. My aim was that you would come away feeling empowered and able to speed your way through your routine in the mornings, while also feeling able to switch off and care for yourself when things get too manic.

One last reminder: ageing is an absolute privilege. There is a confidence that comes with living longer. We're all too aware that we are changing superficially on the outside, and you could probably tell me exactly where each freckle and dimple sits on your face, even with your eyes closed. As I'm learning, joy and peace come when you realise that you know yourself that well on the *inside*, too. We grow as we age. Over the years, I've learned that if I'm ever unsure, I hold the answer within. Be confident in your gut. You got this. Whatever it is.

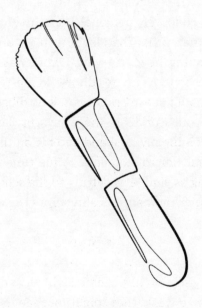

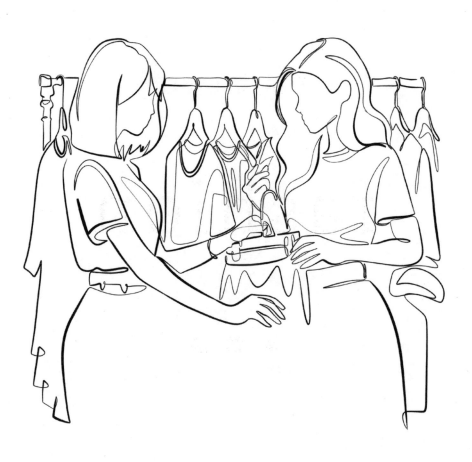

- part two -

fashion

...

Fashion brings me such joy. It's my creative outlet. I was never the most intelligent kid in the crowd but if I was wearing an outfit I loved, it filled me with confidence and made me feel more powerful. I want to teach you how your clothes can do that for you, too, in the most time-efficient and sustainable way possible. I want to help demystify fashion, redefine your wardrobe and perfect your personal style.

If the thought of this all sounds overwhelming, I hear you! But each of the tips and tricks I'll share in this section are succinct, easy to adapt – whatever your lifestyle, shape or size – and can be implemented gradually, rather than all in one go. I want to make sure that once you finish reading these fashion chapters, you feel empowered and in control of your wardrobe and your style, so that one (huge) thing has been ticked off your everyday mental load.

These fashion chapters don't need to be read all in one go, and you can refer back to relevant sections whenever you are ready to tackle them (in particular, the clear-out!).

Let's get started.

Gemma x

- 5 -

start with a wardrobe clear-out

They always say you should tackle the hardest task on your to-do list first, which is why we're kicking things off with the clear-out!

You can't see exactly what you have and what you are working with until you do a cleanse. This chapter will teach you exactly how to clear out what you don't need from your wardrobe – and how to put back what is wearable, useful and practical. It's not about just throwing it back in; if everything slots into its correct place, then you will have a fully functioning wardrobe that will suit your lifestyle and make it quicker and easier to get dressed in the morning, whether you are a busy career woman with back-to-back meetings and no time for procrastinating over what to wear, or a stay-at-home mum who wants to get out of the rut of throwing on leggings and a T-shirt every day.

A clear-out can seem overwhelming to begin with, but the results are so beneficial in the long term. This chapter will teach you about the importance of categories, colour coordination and storage. And the best part is that you don't need to spend a penny while doing it.

A Wardrobe Full of Clothes but Nothing to Wear

How often have you said, 'I've got nothing to wear,' while standing in front of a wardrobe full of clothes? The truth is, we all have plenty to wear, and could probably go through life without ever buying something new again. But when it's all shoved into your wardrobe, you just can't see any of it clearly, or work out how to put it together. It's the same as having a fridge full of ingredients, but no meals. You need to think of the meal (the final outfit), take out all the ingredients (the individual items of clothing) and then combine them together with a recipe (the tips in this book!).

Organising your wardrobe is the first step towards working out exactly what you have to wear and what you are missing, and it's also a really helpful thing to do if you are short on space. This process requires an upfront investment of time, but it will save you time and energy in the long run. The job of organising your wardrobe can seem overwhelming, but if you do it in stages, it can actually be quite therapeutic. Get some girlfriends over or put on a podcast, and work your way through it, section by section.

Take Everything Out

For each section in your wardrobe, from summer dresses to socks, remove every single item (you can do this in stages if doing it all at once is too overwhelming). Give the wardrobe a wipe down, and leave the doors and drawers open to let in some air.

Once everything is out, divide it into the following piles.

To keep

This pile should be made up of items you love, feel great in and wear often: clothes that are comfortable and can easily be styled and incorporated with other pieces in your wardrobe. I don't believe in rules like, 'If you haven't worn it in the last x weeks, it has to go.' Some pieces are special, and you may not have had the right occasion to wear them. If you have any clothes that you love but are one or two sizes too big or too small for you right now, then pop them into a storage bag and place them somewhere else for the time being. The 'to keep' pile is just for current pieces that fit in with you and your lifestyle.

To think about

This pile is for items you don't have anything to wear with, or pieces you aren't sure about. You'll come back to this pile at the end and see if any outfits can be made with your new edited wardrobe, or if there is a gap in your wardrobe for any of these pieces.

To pack away

If an item of clothing is for the wrong season, then box it up. Before you store your seasonal clothes, you need to wash and dry them properly. If it's winter, then pack up your swimsuits and high-summer dresses, and in the summer, pack away your thick jumpers, tights and thermals. The clothes need to be in an airtight container, and I recommend popping in a dryer sheet or lavender sachets to keep things smelling fresh. Don't be tempted to use vacuum bags; they are okay for a couple of weeks or so, but not for storing things for months at a time. When you vacuum-pack clothes, it causes them to wrinkle and they might lose their shape. Don't pack them in cardboard boxes, either, as they can soak up humidity and may become mouldy. Once you are all packed up, the containers can be stored under your bed, in your kids' wardrobes or in a storage cupboard.

To sell

This pile is for items that you don't want to keep but are in great condition, as you could make money by selling them on resale sites or hire sites (see pages 168–174).

To mend

This pile is for items that have mendable holes, or hems that need altering.

To chuck

Any items that have holes in them that can't be repaired or stains that can't be washed out need to go in this pile. It's for items that are no longer wearable.

To pass on

This pile is for items that are in good condition but that you don't think would sell – or for anything you just don't have time or capacity to sell. Give these pieces to friends and family, or donate them to charity.

Categories and Colours

Everything that made the 'to keep' pile now needs to be placed back in the wardrobe in order. The easiest way to plan your wardrobe edit is to use clothing categories, that will then be further organised by colour. Take dresses, for example: you'll place all the dresses together in your wardrobe, starting with the lightest coloured dresses on the left and working your way towards the darkest colour on the right. This means that when you are in a hurry, you'll be able to find exactly what you need quickly. You want your wardrobe to work for you and be arranged as conveniently as possible, as this will help save you time that you probably don't have.

I'm a huge believer in using compartments and containers for storage. Everything needs its own home. This makes it easier to keep things organised and tidy. You don't need to spend lots of money on fancy boxes (although if budget allows, then there is no harm in making it all aesthetically pleasing!). You can use old shoe boxes to store belts, or old Tupperwares to keep your socks in, and you can even cut up your Amazon boxes (yes, we all definitely have them arriving on our doorsteps regularly!) to make dividers for your underwear drawers.

The best hangers are the thin velvet ones. They take up the least space, and their soft, round edges help to stop any damage to your clothes. You don't need to spend a fortune on them; the cheaper versions do the same job. Make sure all the hangers face the same way so they don't get tangled up when you're taking things in and out of your wardrobe.

Storing Shoes and Accessories

How to store your shoes and accessories is hugely dependent on space, but ideally they should be stored inside a cupboard, away from light and dust.

Shoes

The best place for shoes is on shelves behind closed doors. If they are left out, they are more likely to gather dust. Although it's very un-Carrie Bradshaw, you shouldn't store shoes in their cardboard boxes. The cardboard can be susceptible to moisture and humidity, which can cause damage and mould. If you are short on wardrobe space in your bedroom, then think of other places shoes could be stored. I keep all my trainers inside a sideboard in the hallway outside my kitchen (I'm pretty sure said sideboard was intended for storing plates and cups!). I keep my heels in the wardrobe in my bedroom, while my summer sandals are in a drawer under the bed. When it comes to tall boots, I roll up old magazines and insert them to help them hold their shape.

Hats, scarves and bags

Hats, scarves and bags should be stored in boxes, and again, these should ideally be stored in your wardrobe. Try putting these boxes on the shelves at the top; that way, you can just pull down the box you need.

Jewellery

You can get lots of different styles of organisers and compartments for storing jewellery. For necklaces, you can buy specific jewellery hangers with several forward-facing hooks. This way they all drape down and don't get tangled. If this doesn't work for you, then you could lay jewellery trays at the bottom of your wardrobe and just pull out each tray as you need it. You don't need to use a specially made jewellery tray; you could just use any tray and lay down a piece of fabric for the jewellery to be placed on.

To Hang or to Fold?

A general rule of thumb when deciding whether you should hang or fold an item is as follows: if it's a heavier fabric, then fold it; if it easily creases, hang it. Here is a guide on what works best, although of course this depends on the space you have available.

Jeans: Fold on shelves or hang

Jeans are generally made of the thickest fabric out of all the items in your wardrobe, so will hold their shape the best. Folding will generally save space, and give you more room for the items that need to hang. However, if you are short on folding space, these will last just as well if they are hung up.

Trousers: Hang

The fabric of trousers is usually lighter, so it's best to drape them over a hanger so they hold their shape.

Dresses: Hang

Generally, anything made from a more flowy fabric that has movement (silk, chiffon, linen, etc.) should be hung up so it can breathe. If you have a knitted dress, or a very heavy dress, then it's best to fold it.

Blouses: Hang

The rule above for dresses also applies to blouses: if it would move about if the wind blew, then it should be hung. This will cause fewer creases.

Skirts: Hang (using clip hangers)

Hanging skirts makes it easier to see what is in your wardrobe.

T-shirts: Fold on shelves or in drawers

Arrange T-shirts by colour and style. Keep all your vests together in one place, then short-sleeved T-shirts in another, long-sleeved T-shirts in another, and so on. This way, you can grab what you are looking for quickly.

Knitwear: Fold on shelves

Never hang knitwear; this will cause it to very quickly lose its shape and stretch.

Underwear: Fold in drawers

Use drawer dividers to keep your underwear drawers neat. Place your bras together, ideally in colour order, then use the dividers to separate pants and socks.

Outerwear: Hang

Folding coats and similar items will take up unnecessary space, and can ruin their shape.

Mind the Gaps

Once everything is placed back in your wardrobe in its correct place, it will be easier for you to identify any gaps, and work out what extras you need to complete your wardrobe (if any – remember, you probably don't *need* to buy anything). This wardrobe detox allows you to see clearly what is missing, and you'll also be able to see what you have lots of (hands up if it's a Breton top!), which may help you get a clear idea of what your personal style is. If you do feel like you need something, then make a note of what is missing so that the next time you see your favourite shop or brand holding a sale, you can make a precise, deliberate purchase, rather than wasting cash on something you don't need. In the next chapter there are tips and advice on how to identify your own style, and this will also help you to spot any gaps.

■ ■ ■

Hopefully you've now learned how to organise your wardrobe space so that you can clearly see what you have. Many people find this process quite cathartic! A reminder, though: this process doesn't need to happen all in one go. If you find it too much, then just focus on one section per week. Perhaps start with your jumpers, then plan some time the following weekend to go through your dresses, then your skirts, and so on. Even sorting the dreaded pyjama shelf will feel amazing once it's been done. And no, you don't need that T-shirt that you've had for twenty years and is full of holes. I know it's comfy to sleep in, but enough's enough – time for it to go!

- 6 -

discover your personal style and build a capsule wardrobe

Now that you have cleared out the clutter and can see exactly what you have, it's time to start the process of identifying your personal style. Once you've fully established your personal style, we'll look at some guidance on key items that you can use to tailor your wardrobe to suit it, including my wardrobe non-negotiables.

Finding Your Personal Style

Discovering your personal style can be tricky. You may feel like you just like loads of different pieces of clothing, or that you don't tend to favour a particular style. Alternatively, you may find that you do the opposite, and only wear one style of clothing all the time. You may have bought pieces that are still hanging in your wardrobe with the tags on, because you never worked out what they go with or how to make them work. Figuring out your personal style is important, as it will stop you buying pieces that you don't need, and will help you invest in the items you will get most use out of.

After working in the fashion industry for all these years and styling hundreds of women, I don't believe that there is one clear-cut way to define your personal style. There are a few different things that could help, and by doing some of these (or a little bit of all of them) you'll soon be able to see a pattern forming of the things you like.

A wardrobe cleanse

Removing everything from your wardrobe, assessing what you own, culling what you don't like and keeping what you love can help reveal what your style is.

Take a closer look

Set some time aside to properly look at clothes. Don't buy anything, but go browsing in a store or online. Take photos or screenshots of all the things you come across that you love. Keep an eye on them over a period of time (at least a couple of weeks), and think about how they would work with other items you own, and where you'd wear them. You may find that you end up deleting some of the pictures. Our fast-paced lives make us think that if we like something initially, we need it immediately, so this method helps to slow down your fashion decisions. As you curate the photos or screenshots into a mood board of pieces you love, a pattern will begin to form.

Mood boarding

To take the step above further, start collating images of outfits you like; these might be photos of yourself in favourite items, shots of a particular outfit on a celebrity, or someone you follow on Instagram whose style you admire. You could use Pinterest, create a style inspiration folder on your phone, or physically print out the images and stick them onto card. You may find with this method that you actually already own some of the pieces on your mood board, but now you'll have new ways to style them.

The three-word method

You may have heard of this technique as it's been very popular on social media over the last year or so but it's actually been around for a really long time. Simply think of three adjectives you'd use to describe your style; for example, Sam would use 'practical, classic and muted' and my three words would be 'leopard, unconventional and unpolished.' (Could we be any more different?) Every time you make a purchase, you need to check if it fits in with at least one of your three words. This is a great method, and it makes it easier to shop if you've narrowed down your categories. Fashion stylist and writer Alexandra Fullerton has taken it one step further and launched a website called My3Words.co which is a handy tool to help you find clothing based on your three words. Alex says that she is still attracted to clothes because they look good but will leave them on the shelf because they don't chime with her words. She often uses the analogy of interiors: 'You might see a cushion or a vase in the shops but if it doesn't go with your decor, you'll walk away. We should do that more often with our wardrobes.'

Don't follow trends

This is so important. As young kids, we were always taught that just because someone else liked something, it didn't mean that we had to like it also (did anyone else's parents constantly say, 'If so-and-so jumped off a cliff, would you?'!). So when new trends are announced at the beginning of each season, it would be crazy if we all liked all of them. Don't buy something just because everyone else has it; only buy it if you absolutely love it and it works with other things you own. I research the trends each season as part of my job, and it's really hard not to get sucked into something because you see it everywhere, but following trends won't help you define your own personal style; it will only encourage you to copy someone else's.

Have a try-on session

Put together outfits that you own and properly try them on, with the correct shoes and all! It may be time-consuming (get some girlfriends over and make a night of it), but it's so worth it. It's easier to see how something fits when it's on your body. Take pictures of the outfits you love, get rid of the ones you don't. Then look through all the photos of the ones that made the cut, and you should see a pattern of what your style is.

Once you've worked it out, remember that it doesn't *always* need a label. We don't need to define ourselves as 'bohemian' or 'girly' or 'seventies' in order to make wise purchases. The whole purpose of defining your style is so that you shop better; if a label helps you do that, then so be it, but if you can't quite put your finger on a word to describe it, then all that really matters is that you shop wisely. Buy clothes that you love, that make you feel good, and that you look forward to putting on. You need to have a wardrobe that you enjoy wearing, not one that you stare at feeling uninspired.

TIM new purchase questionnaire

Before making any purchases, it's always worth asking yourself the questions below, because it's so easy to get caught up in thinking you need something new.

1. Do I really need the item? (We very rarely actually *need* something.)
2. Do I really love the item and feel great in it?
3. Do I own anything similar that does the same job?
4. Does it fit in with my personal style?
5. Can I make more than three outfits with it?
6. Can I style it with pieces I already own?
7. Will it help me get dressed quicker?
8. Is it well made, so that it will last a long time?
9. Does it fit properly, or will it need to be altered?
10. If it wasn't on sale, would I still want to buy it?

Building a Capsule Wardrobe

Once you've worked out exactly what your personal style is, you need to build your wardrobe around it. Capsule wardrobes are a great way to start doing this. A capsule wardrobe is the bones of your wardrobe; the pieces you'll have at the core of what you wear. Everyone's capsule wardrobe will look slightly different, as you have to make it work for you, your job and your lifestyle. Usually, each piece in a capsule wardrobe can be mixed and matched with the others to create multiple outfits, and once you've got the capsule sorted, you can add extra pieces that suit you and define your personality. It's so important to include pieces that make you look and feel confident, and if that means rotating lots of pieces that are similar in style, then that is okay. It might feel repetitive, but if you have a stylish 'uniform' that is personal to you, it will make it easier and quicker to get dressed in the morning.

Here is a rough guide to the items that are useful to have so that you can build outfits quickly and easily. If you live in the UK, then quite a few pieces can be overlapped from autumn to summer. There is probably no need to buy anything new as you create your capsule wardrobe, especially now you've had a wardrobe cleanse. Most of these items will already exist in your wardrobe in some form, and you don't need everything on this list. There will be some pieces that fit in with your personal style, and others that you'd just never wear. For me, it's the trench; it's often considered a staple in a capsule wardrobe, but I'm just not a trench gal. A trench wouldn't work with the rest of my wardrobe, and I don't find them practical (I'm either sweating or shivering, no in-between!). However, a trench might work really well for you and be a useful item. Everyone is different, so pick and choose what works for you.

Autumn/winter (A/W) capsule wardrobe

Tops: Breton striped long-sleeved T-shirt, black cami, neutral T-shirts, denim shirt, casual logo sweatshirt

Trousers: Blue jeans, black jeans, leather trousers, tailored trousers, leggings

Jackets: Leather jacket, neutral blazer, trench, black blazer

Shoes: Heeled boots, flat boots, trainers, smart flats (loafers), strappy heels

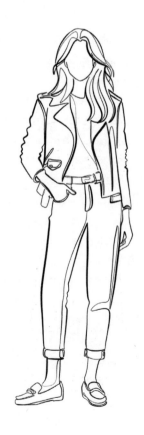

Spring/summer (S/S) capsule wardrobe

Tops: Breton striped short-sleeved T-shirt, neutral vests, neutral T-shirts, denim shirt, white linen shirt, smart blouse

Trousers: Lightweight tailored trousers, lightweight casual trousers, white jeans, blue jeans, cropped black trousers

Dresses: Failsafe black summer dress, printed dress (perhaps floral or leopard, depending on your style)

Shoes: Smart flats (loafers), chunky sandals, barely there sandals, low-rise non-chunky trainers (like Converse, Adidas Gazelle or Nike), strappy heels

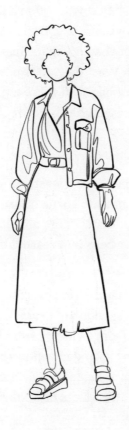

Accessories

As with many of the pieces that help shape and mould your wardrobe, your accessories will depend on your personal style and lifestyle. Your accessories (bags, belts, hats, jewellery and sunglasses) can all overlap within your A/W and S/S wardrobes, and if you shop wisely, they can all be used throughout the year, apart from the odd piece like a straw-style summer bag, or raffia belts.

Bags

If anyone ever asks me what it's worth spending their birthday money on, I always say bags. It is *always* worth investing in bags. Even if your body fluctuates in size, a bag will always fit you! There is no reason why a good-quality handbag shouldn't last you a lifetime if you treat it with care. It makes much more sense to splash out/save up/ask Santa for one well-made bag, rather than going for high-street bags that you'll have to replace year after year. They don't have the same quality of craftsmanship as a luxury bag. And if luxury is out of the question, at least go for real leather, as it has much more longevity compared to synthetics.

Belts

Again, plastic/synthetic belts are a waste of money, as the plastic peels pretty quickly. You don't need to spend a fortune on belts, however, and you really don't need that many. There are lots of high-street brands that have brilliant leather belts at a reasonable price.

Jewellery

I've always stuck to the mantra 'No rules for jewels'. Grab something in the supermarket clothes section when stocking up on veg; pick up some costume jewellery from a charity shop for £2; have a rummage at a car-boot sale on a sunny spring morning; scour eBay for luxury brands at a bargain price; or wear your best gold or finest diamonds. Go chunky or delicate. Layer necklaces or hoop earrings. Combine gold and silver, or stick to one metal. Whatever takes your fancy. There are so many brilliant options out there. Gold-plated jewellery (where a thin layer of liquid gold is plated over another metal) can be really affordable and look very effective. So simple, so quick, but so effective. Building a jewellery collection is a must if you want to look put together. Jewellery can add personality and life to a really simple outfit. It doesn't need to be a luxury, and you really don't need to spend much money on it to have an impact

The four capsule wardrobe non-negotiables

If we take a deeper dive into the capsule wardrobe, there are a few non-negotiable items in there. These are pieces of clothing that you can throw together when you've had three hours of sleep, and only have three minutes to get ready but want and need to look like you have your sh*t together.

1. Great-fitting denim

There's no point having twenty pairs of jeans but only wearing the one pair that you actually like and feel good in. Have a cull. Pass the old pairs on to charity, give them to a friend, or sell them on eBay or Vinted. If they are too damaged for wear, take them to a Traid recycling bin. Traid is a network of over 1,500 locations in the UK where you can drop unwanted clothes for recycling so that they don't end up in landfill.

Don't just stick to classic blue jeans. Mix it up with cropped wide-legged denim to balance out your body shape, or try a pair that have embellishment or other details on them to highlight your best features. Just make sure you own jeans that make you feel good, and that you look forward to wearing. When you find denim that you LOVE, then bulk-buy. Grab a couple of pairs of your favourite style, in the same or different shades, so that you can alternate and make them last longer.

Jeans should always be a really snug fit when you first try them on, so they then mould with your body. If they feel too comfortable in the first try-on session, then they will end up going baggy. I used to make sure my personal styling clients had to do an awkward dance to get into their denim; if it didn't feel awkward, then jeans were a size too big. If they *feel* too tight on your waist but fit everywhere else and you are in a rush, then you can always slightly wet the waist, as this will cause them to loosen quickly so they're more comfortable.

Don't put your jeans in the dryer. The heat damages the elasticity. They might feel tighter momentarily, but they will quickly become very loose. Always air-dry them.

I don't think it's ever worth spending much on denim; the great British high-street does denim so well. Stores worth looking at for great denim in a vast size range, with multiple leg lengths and different styles, include:

- Abercrombie: UK 4–26, three leg lengths
- Boden: UK 4–24, four leg lengths
- Hush: UK 4–18, three leg lengths
- Levi's: UK 4–24, three leg lengths

When purchasing jeans, you must always check the label to see the fabric composition. Most jeans have a percentage of elastane in them. Too much elastane, and they will be thin denim and skin-tight; too little elastane and they'll be thick denim, meaning they'll stretch out and never hold their shape. Denim that's 100 per cent cotton will always lose its shape because there's no stretch in the fabric, so the cotton threads expand and, once expanded, they won't ever go back to their original size. If you go for 100 per cent cotton jeans, choose a baggy or boyfriend-style that doesn't require them to be fitted or to hold their shape. Ideally, you want a combination of 98 per cent cotton and 2 per cent elastane; this means the jeans won't have much give, but will still be comfortable.

2. Leather jacket

A totally timeless item. Buy well, and you will have it for ever. A leather jacket can be worn on a cool summer evening, thrown over a strappy dress, or layered up in winter with a hooded jumper underneath and a big coat on top. I recommend only buying real leather, as otherwise it will look cheap, and you will need to replace it often as the plastic won't last (it tends to wear away over the elbows first.) Go down a size if it is even the slightest bit big, because real leather will stretch. It's best to stick with black so that it goes with everything. I have a real leather jacket that I bought when I first started working as a stylist for Topshop in 2006. I remember spending my wages on it, using my staff discount and panicking about how much it cost at the time! It's now sixteen years old and I still wear it often. It's worn and moulded in the most beautiful, natural way. All Saints has always been a leather jacket haven; they have so many different styles and shapes that it's worth going into a store to try on a few so you can figure out which shape you like best.

3. Jewellery

Throughout history, jewellery has been used to signify many different things, from wealth to religion to creative expression. Today, it's just as important as ever.

Personally, jewellery is my main non-negotiable. My mum built up her own vintage jewellery brand, Susan Caplan, by herself from scratch when my sisters and I were young, and this had a huge impact on how my future was shaped. She used to drag us around car boot sales, eyes peeled for an original art deco Napier necklace or Trifari earrings from the 1930s, which she'd snap up to sell on. Her eye for spotting vintage Chanel in excellent condition is second to none, a life skill that I hope I inherit!

Jewellery defines my personal style. I just counted, and I have fourteen pieces of jewellery that I wear 24/7. I sleep and shower wearing them. From stacked earrings in my eight piercings, to layered necklaces and rings, my jewellery is so personal to me, and I feel naked without it. Some are just cheap pieces I've picked up over the years. I have a tiny diamond ring on my thumb that my mum found in a vintage store in Glasgow for £10. Some of my jewellery signifies memorable moments in my life, to do with my children or my marriage. All of them are sentimental, and all have a story behind them.

The right jewellery will instantly pull an outfit together and make it look styled. Jewellery can make you feel more confident and powerful, and is a way to show your personality or make a statement, with very little effort involved.

4. A basic T-shirt collection

You don't need to spend much money to look effortless quickly, and that's certainly the case when it comes to basics. Your wardrobe should hold two black, two white and two grey T-shirts (you can build on these colours further once you've established your personal style and know what you'd wear daily). A great T-shirt should be 100 per cent cotton (ideally organic cotton). I try to avoid synthetic fabrics like polyester at all costs; they are essentially made from plastic, and as well as being awful for our planet, they will also make you sweat more as they aren't natural fabrics, so aren't breathable.

Go for a T-shirt with a slightly wider ribbed collar (this always looks more premium), and make sure the sleeves aren't too tight. Cos, Arket and & Other Stories do great basics for a really reasonable price.

Shoes

Whether you own four pairs of shoes or 400, we all need footwear that will be functional and fit in with our lifestyle (she says, while glancing at her wardrobe containing 108 pairs of heels that rarely get worn!).

There are six styles of shoes that everyone should own in order to have a fully kitted-out wardrobe, and to have something that will work for all occasions. If budget allows, then you can expand on each style with multiples.

- smart flats (loafers/ballet shoes)
- flat boots
- trainers (fashionable, rather than functional for wardrobe-building purposes)
- heeled boots
- strappy heels
- summer sandals

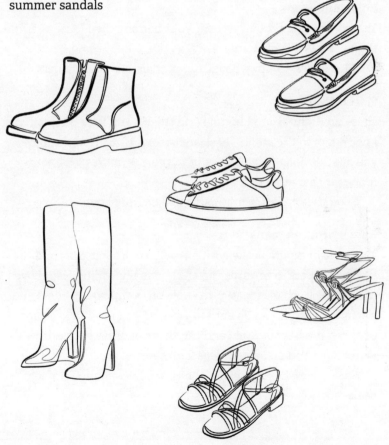

The denim and footwear guide

If I had a pound for every time someone asked me which shoes work best with certain denim, I'd be lying on a sun lounger in my Mallorcan villa overlooking the sea, accepting a drink from my butler while dripping in Chanel! Once you've worked out what your go-to denim shape is, then it's time to identify the shoe shapes that are most flattering with these jeans.

Boyfriend jeans
These jeans are more fitted over your bottom, then loose over the thighs. They straighten out towards the ankle.

Shoe styles: Chunky boots, flat sandals, slimline trainers

Flared jeans
These are tight around bottom and thighs, and flare out from the knee down to the ankle. These are best worn with heels unless you are tall/ long-legged. Lean in to their seventies look with footwear that suits that style.

Shoe styles: Platform heels, heeled chunky boots

Barrel or mom jeans
This style of denim is always high-waisted. It's loose around the leg, then tapers in towards the ankle, usually ending just above ankle, which makes it easier to show off your shoes. Unless you are tall, this style can be hard to wear, as you need to keep space between the hem of jeans and the shoes in order to not drown your shape and make your legs look shorter.

Shoe styles: Loafers, ballet shoes, sandals, slimline trainers, heels, boots (tucked in)

Straight jeans

These jeans are straight from waist to ankle. They can be a slim cut (more fitted) or a looser fit (a baggier style), but the shape is always the same.

Shoe styles: Full-length – loafers, slim trainers, sandals, heels. Cropped – loafers, boots, slim trainers, chunky trainers, sandals, heels

Skinny jeans

Jeans that are fitted all the way down, from waist to ankle.

Shoe styles: Loafers, chunky or slim trainers, sandals, chunky boots, heels, knee-high boots

Underwear

Underwear is a basic necessity of life. It's also important when it comes to building outfits, because it can help hold you in at the correct place, smooth out an area you don't want to focus on, create or enhance your desired shape, or give you an added layer of confidence.

Here are ten things worth bearing in mind when sorting through your underwear drawer:

1. You shouldn't ever be able to feel your underwear when wearing it. Comfort is key.
2. There is no need to ever own a white bra. It will never stay as white as the first day you bought it, and it will always show through whatever you are wearing.
3. If you don't want your underwear to show through something white or sheer, then match your undies to your skin tone, not to

the piece of clothing. I have some skin-tone knickers for when I'm pale, and another shade for when I have a bit of a tan.

4. Everyone should own one matching set. It's a real confidence-booster.

5. There are no rules for the pants you need to own. Don't like wearing thongs? Don't buy them.

6. Seam-free underwear actually works – & Other Stories do a brilliant pair of high-waisted, seam-free knickers that don't show through.

7. Wearing the right-sized bra is important for posture and comfort, and there are so many places you can go to for a free fitting. Marks & Spencer have a great and easy-to-use online bra-fitting tool, and Bravissimo has a helpful online guide.

8. According to Stripe & Stare (one of the comfiest, sustainable underwear brands on the high street) there has been a decrease in thong sales. Katie Lopes, co-founder and Creative and Sustainability director says, 'Our thong sales used to represent 20 per cent of our underwear sales and it is now less than 6 per cent. In turn we cannot keep up with the demand for our high rise!' So, ladies, don't forget – comfort is key!

9. Control underwear is great, not only if you are conscious of certain areas on your body, but also to smooth out indents and joins in your garments.

10. Treat your underwear with care. Ideally handwash it, but if that isn't possible, then always wash your bras in a laundry bag on a cool wash. This helps them keep their shape, and will stop the hooks from snagging on other clothes in the machine.

The underwear directory

The brand that focuses on inclusivity and body positivity: Skims
Don't let the fact that a Kardashian started this brand put you off.
It offers underwear solutions for all shapes and sizes, and includes
underwear and shapewear. The technically constructed shapewear can
stretch to two times its size, making it genuinely comfortable to wear.
Skims offer a huge size range , with underwear and shapewear in sizes
XXS to 4XL, and bras in sizes 30A to 46H.

The brand that caters for all shades of nude: Nubian Skin
As mentioned above, it's important that your underwear matches your
skin tone, rather than your clothes, and for so long, for so many
women of colour, that has been almost impossible. Nubian Skin have
changed that. They have a super-handy colour-matching guide that
allows you to select which celeb's skin tone is most similar to yours,
and then suggests the bra colour you should choose. Nubian Skin also
launched the UK's first softie breast forms for mastectomy patients of
colour, and even did the undies for Beyoncé's Formation World Tour.
If that's not enough of an accreditation, then I don't know what is!
Sizes 30A–40HH.

The brand that cares about the planet: Stripe & Stare
Struggling to find knickers that sit somewhere between overly sexy
and frumpy? Introducing Stripe & Stare, a female-founded, British
underwear brand that is committed to sustainability by producing
knickers that are quite literally made from trees. According to their
website, the fabric they use is 'three times softer than cotton, wears
better and is just as breathable as fresh air in a forest of responsibly
planted trees'. They have a knicker shape to suit most needs. I wear
them most days and can confirm that they are so soft and
comfortable. Sizes UK 6–22

The brand that is more inclusive than you think: Victoria's Secret

In 2021, Victoria's Secret announced that they were rebranding. It was a very welcome rebrand, as they had lost so much cultural credibility, but we believe in second chances – and safe to say, they've made huge changes. They've kept some of their sex appeal, but now it comes with a side of functionality, and the brand has become way more inclusive than it was when it comes to body diversity. Most (not all) bras now come in sizes 30AA to 44DD, and they have a great selection of multifunctional bras if you are looking for something that works with an awkward-shaped top or dress. They offer free in-store fitting appointments, where you can bring in an outfit and their stylists will help find an underwear solution for it – no appointment necessary.

The brand we all know and love: Marks & Spencer

Ahh, good old trusty M&S. No doubt the place you went with your mum to pick out your first bra. They went through a phase where they lost their cool, but it is now back with a vengeance. You can book a free bra-fitting appointment at your local store online, or follow their online guide. They are size-inclusive with a brilliant price point, and offer pregnancy and mastectomy ranges.

Swimwear

As I've got older, I've realised the importance of investing in swimwear. Gone are the days where I'd do an ASOS haul of cheap and cheerful bikinis that I'd wear for one summer, only to find that the fabric had stretched and gone see-through, or the colours had faded out. I've now established the shape of swimwear that I feel good in and feel happy to put on when I arrive on holiday. I want to create curves and shape, as

I'm pretty straight up and down (otherwise known as a rectangle body shape), so I go for a slightly higher leg (not *Love Island* high!), as this elongates my short legs and creates more waist definition. I wear a thin strap (tan lines) and keep prints, patterns, ruffles or bow details on top to draw attention there, which keeps my silhouette more balanced. Finding the right shape of swimwear for you can be empowering and can boost your confidence. A lot of it is trial and error, but in the brand directory below, I've included some guidance as to what might suit your shape best.

Choosing swimwear can be pretty daunting for most, so it's worth owning two or three brilliant-fitting swimsuits or bikinis that you feel good in, rather than ten that don't fit well and will fall apart after chasing your kid around a pool, or splashing about on a girls' weekend away. (Side note: I'm a huge fan of a pre-holiday spray tan. It gives instant confidence for when you arrive on the beach, it fades naturally because you moisturise it each time you apply SPF, and it never goes patchy. By the time it fades on day three or four, a natural tan has usually developed, so my pasty Scottish skin isn't as pasty!)

The swimwear directory

The long-lasting brand: Hunza G
The British brand Hunza was originally founded in 1984. Thirty-seven years later, it was brought back to life and rebranded as Hunza G. This carbon-neutral company use 9,953,280 stitches in every swimsuit, so that they always go back to their original shape after being worn. They come in one size, which fits roughly size UK 6–16, and can be worn in pregnancy also. The darker-coloured fabrics are a better investment than the lighter shades, as when the fabric stretches out, the paler shades can go thinner in some areas and look a little see-through. Sam and I own more Hunzas than should be allowed!

The brand to choose if you are tall, petite or somewhere in the middle: Boden

Boden's swimwear sits at the higher end of the high street, but most of their designs come in regular, petite and tall. They offer sizes UK 6–22, and their swimwear comes in a huge variety of prints and patterns. Some designs also have a cup size so you can work out the correct fit for your shape.

The brand to choose if you like prints, patterns and bold colour: Solid & Striped

A personal favourite of mine, their offerings are full of beautiful prints, patterns and bold colours. They have a handy tool on their website where you can shop by fit, such as 'full coverage' or 'underwire' or 'low-rise', which eliminates the need to spend hours scrolling for exactly what you're after. Most of their prints come in numerous styles so you can mix and match depending on your favourite shape. They also have a fit guide on their website with women of various shapes and sizes wearing the swimwear so you can see it all clearly.

The brand for bigger busts: Curvy Kate

Curvy Kate offer swimwear in cup sizes D–K and back sizes 28–44. They have really useful bra-fitting videos on their website, which can also be used for swimwear, and a huge range of swimsuits and bikinis. The range can be overwhelming, so use their filters to narrow it down by picking your preferred style, size and colour.

The sustainable brand: Prism

This brand has been going strong for over ten years, but in 2019 they developed a range called PRISM^2, which has sustainability at the forefront. The swimwear is dyed using a Greenpeace-certified technique, and the factory used to create them has a Higg Index certification (this is a tool that measures the value of sustainability). Each item in the PRISM^2 collection can be worn as swimwear, underwear or sportswear. The brand comes in sizes UK 6–24.

The small business: Tona
A UK-based sustainable swimwear brand founded by stylist Tona Stell, offering sizes UK 8–20. Their printed swimwear uses Econyl, which is a type of nylon made using items that would otherwise end up in landfill. It's particularly great for bikinis and swimsuits, as it is more resistant to chlorine and SPF than other fabrics. All the packaging is recycled and recyclable, and the fabrics are even sent over by boat to reduce greenhouse gas emissions.

The high-street brand: & Other Stories
If budget doesn't allow you to spend on a higher price-point brand, & Other Stories has a great range of swimwear. The key is getting in there early, as it's usually all sold out by the time summer is in full swing. Make your purchases by May at the latest to ensure you have your pick of the range. They do a great selection of textures, prints and patterns in a range of shapes and styles, from classic pieces to more fashion-forward looks, and all at a really reasonable price.

■ ■ ■

People often talk about fashion being superficial, but it can be so empowering to establish exactly how you will present yourself and how that makes you feel on the inside. By this point, I hope you are feeling more confident with your wardrobe, how it's set out, what your own personal style is and the essential items that can help elevate your outfits.

- 7 -

dressing for your body shape

First things first, body shape and size are two completely different things. You can have a petite hourglass shape and wear a size 6 or a size 26. Sometimes when trying on clothes, you might find that a particular piece of clothing doesn't sit right, and this issue can usually be fixed with a couple of tiny tweaks. This chapter is going to teach you how to establish what your own body shape is, and this will enable you to work out the most flattering outfits for your body, and how those tiny tweaks can have a big impact.

Body Shapes Through History

The earliest example of a portrayal of a woman's shape is found in the *Venus of Willendorf*, a statue from somewhere between 24,000 and 22,000 BCE. It is one of the oldest works of art in existence. It portrays the woman's shape with a large bust, a fuller stomach and curvaceous legs. There have been suggestions that she represents fertility or a mother goddess, but perhaps it was just a representation of a woman in the Palaeolithic times. The statue is on display in the Natural History Museum in Vienna, in case you happen to find yourself nearby and need a reminder of how fabulous and diverse all bodies are.

As a society, we've been fascinated by size and the ideal body type for centuries, and this 'ideal' has changed throughout the years. The changes have usually been to do with whoever is the prominent female actress, star, or 'it' girl of the moment. In the 1910s, for example, the 'Gibson Girl' aesthetic was celebrated – an hourglass shape with a cinched-in waist – while the 1920s were all about a boyish frame with no curves. In the 1930s, fuller shapes came into fashion, and then the 1940s celebrated the pin-up girl with cone-shaped bras (can't imagine that becoming a mainstream trend again!). As time moved on, the 1950s focused on a Jessica Rabbit shape, with curves being ultra prominent. There were even ads for supplements to help slimmer women gain weight so they could try to achieve this shape. In the 1960s and 1970s, there was a shift towards the slimline shape of people like Twiggy, and clothes that could alter your shape (like corsets) were replaced with diets and fitness crazes. The slim-girl aesthetic carried on through the eighties and nineties as the supermodel shape took over, and when Kate Moss became the face of Calvin Klein ads in the 1990s, the term 'waif' gained momentum. This had a psychological impact on many women, who began to believe the media's notion that skinny was best.

In recent times, things seem to be changing. With a focus on body positivity and body confidence, it feels like things have progressed in a positive direction for the first time in a long time. There are so many inspiring women now in the public eye with the most beautiful curves. Catwalk shows these days have so much body diversity (although there is still a long way to go!), and social media means that we can curate our own feeds to show us the shapes and sizes that resonate with us most.

Loving your body is a journey, and might not be something that can happen overnight, but never forget – everyone else is too busy focusing on their own bodies to notice yours! The 'ideal' shapes have changed so much throughout the years, and will continue to do so, so it's really not worth focusing your energy or time on trying to turn yourself into something you are not, especially when that 'something' will inevitably change again. We are born with these bodies for a reason. Yes, you can accentuate the bits you love with clothes and accessories, but what makes our world so wonderful is that no two people are the same – so embrace what you have. Worst-case scenario? Just fake confidence. You might surprise yourself and grow to love it! Comparison is the thief of joy, so try to remember that the 'ideal' body shape for you is the body you live in, and it's up to you to look after it and celebrate it.

Dressing for Your Body Shape

When it comes to dressing for your body shape, a key aspect is creating balanced proportions. Certain lines and shapes can divide your body – or your outfit – into different parts, and much of this comes down to the proportions of your upper and lower body. This is important in terms of styling because different outfit components can work together with your natural frame in order to create what is perceived as the most flattering look.

Women have been told for years to work out what fruit their body resembles in order to find the most flattering cut of jeans (side note – have you ever heard anyone suggest that men do the same?!), and while this is actually a good rule of thumb if you aren't so confident with outfit choices, it's quite an outdated theory, and you must always remember that you should wear what you love, and what makes you feel good, whether your body more closely resembles an apple or pear. Understanding your shape and knowing how to create and build a silhouette that you love can be the basis for great style, but we shouldn't ever 'hide' or 'correct' our shapes, we should celebrate them for what they are and learn how to make the most of them.

How to Measure Your Body

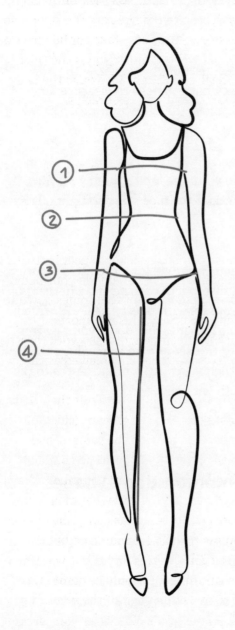

Before working out which shape category you fit into, it's worth taking your measurements. This can help to work out your shape if you are unsure, and it's also useful to have your measurements to hand when shopping online. All brands vary slightly when it comes to sizing, so you can compare your measurements against the brand's sizing guide to check that the item will fit correctly.

It might be helpful to do this with someone helping so you get accurate measurements, but if you struggle with this (or working out your body type), you could always invest in an appointment with a personal shopper or stylist. John Lewis offer a free service, with no obligation to buy. So even if it's just a one-off appointment to get you started, it can be really useful.

1. Chest
Keeping the tape measure parallel with the floor, start with tape on the fullest point of the bust and wrap it around the body.

2. Waist
Put your hands around the smallest part of your waist, with your hands resting on your hips. This is what you need to measure: the narrowest part of your waist, just above the belly button, but below your rib cage.

3. Hips
Stand with your feet together and wrap the tape around your hips, passing it over your bottom. Make sure the tape stays straight all the way around.

4. Inseam
It's worth taking two measurements here: one for more fitted trousers, and one for wide-leg trousers. It's also worth considering whether you are using the measurement for trousers with flats or heels. For fitted trousers where you'd have an ankle gap, measure down your leg from crotch to ankle bone. For wider-leg trousers, or trousers where the hem would almost touch the ground, then measure from the crotch to the flat of your foot. It's best to do both with shoes on.

Five of the Most Common Body Shapes

I'm going to use shapes here, as this is the easiest way to explain it, but how you describe your body is up to you – in this day and age, women don't need to be objectified! You might fit comfortably into one body-shape category, or relate to a mix of two. When working out your body shape, remember that size doesn't matter at all. No matter your dress size, you can be any of the body shapes listed below. It also doesn't matter what shape you are – it is just a useful guide to help you get dressed and make you feel more confident in the process. A useful tip is to find a celebrity or well-known person who has the same body shape as you, and whose personal style you like so that you can take inspiration from them and their wardrobe.

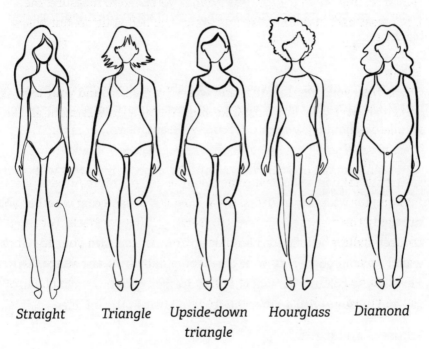

Straight   Triangle   Upside-down   Hourglass   Diamond
                         triangle

Straight

Kate Middleton, Drew Barrymore, Oprah Winfrey, Octavia Spencer, Nicole Kidman

Your hips and shoulders are the same width, and your waist and bust are a similar width. You don't have many curves or particularly go 'in' or 'out' anywhere.

Styling tips for a straight shape

As your upper and lower body are in proportion, it is best to accentuate the waist in order to break up the rectangle. Do this by wearing something high-waisted, or belting in your outfit. You can also add more dimensions to your upper and lower parts by wearing prints, patterns or embellishments, or wearing structured clothes. Wear bright colours top and bottom, broken up in the middle with a black belt.

Tops

Avoid square necks, as this will exaggerate the shape of your body. Instead, stick with a curvy shape like a sweetheart neckline, or go for an off-the-shoulder, V-neck or scoop neck, as this will break up the chest area. When it comes to sleeves, fitted sleeves will add to the rectangular shape of your body, so opt for a loose fit, as this will create the illusion of shape.

Dresses

Dresses should be balanced on the top and bottom, and pulled in at the waist. You can pop a belt on to create the pulled-in waist shape. You can also use colour to create shape in dresses, going for bold colours top and bottom, with a different-coloured belt in the middle.

Trousers and jeans

To add curves to your bottom half, wear flares, bootcut or boyfriend-style loose jeans. Add pockets and pleats to draw attention to the area.

Denim styles to try: High-waisted, skinny, slim-fit, straight-fit, bootcut, wide-leg.

Jackets

Nip your jackets in at the waist or add a belt over the jacket to pull it in if it's a blazer. Wear a belted tie around the waist on coats. Don't wear jackets that end at your waist; make sure they are longer in length to draw the eye downward.

Swimwear
Use frills, prints and patterns, tie-side bikini bottoms or cut-out swimsuits to create curves.

Triangle

Jennifer Lopez, Beyoncé, Kim Kardashian, Rebel Wilson, Rihanna, Kate Winslet

A triangle body shape is narrower at the top and wider at the bottom. You may be more flat-chested with slim arms and a smaller waist, and then have a curvaceous bottom and thighs that are wider than your shoulders.

Styling tips for a triangle shape
Use prints and textures to create extra volume on your torso to draw attention away from your bottom half, and focus on balance. Emphasise your waist.

Tops
To widen the shoulder area, wear short-sleeved T-shirts with loose sleeves, and blouses in bright colours, with floral prints and stripes. A wider, round neckline or off-shoulder top can also create the illusion of widening the shoulder area. Slim-fitting shirts or wrap-over shirts are flattering. Thicker knitwear can add volume to your upper half. Wear items with structured shoulders to visually widen the shoulder line. Don't hide your waistline with longer T-shirts or tops; either wear a cropped length or tuck them in.

Trousers and jeans
Avoid pockets and patterns on your widest area. Flat-fronted, mid- or high-waisted styles are your best bet, as they will hug your waist. Flares can balance out your ankles and hips, so will work well.
   Denim styles to try: Straight, high-rise, flare, bootcut, wide-leg.

Dresses

Choose flowy wrap dresses, or draped dresses that pull in at the waist. Fit-and-flare style dresses are super-flattering, as are A-line dresses, and dresses with V-necks, as these will elongate the top part of your body.

Jackets

Choose cropped jackets that sit at your waist, or longer-line coats with details around the neck, bust or shoulders, like shoulder pads, pockets or embellishments. Don't wear coats or jackets that end at the widest parts of your hips. Focus on shoulder structure and belted waists. Cropped jackets in bright colours will draw the eye upwards. Longer blazers are a really flattering style for triangle body shapes. Trench coats also work well because the belted waist makes space between your upper and lower body, and the shoulder epaulettes draw the eye upwards.

Swimwear

Add volume on your top half to create the illusion of a balanced top and bottom. You can do this by wearing printed tops, frills or ruffles, or wide straps with details and patterns.

Upside-down triangle

Angelina Jolie, Naomi Campbell, Renée Zellweger, Zendaya, Kim Cattrall

You are heavier on top than on the bottom, with broad shoulders, a narrow bust and waist, and slim legs.

Styling tips for upside-down triangle shape

You want to create waist definition and highlight volume on your bottom half so that it balances out with the top half.

Tops

The aim is to make your shoulders look softer, and this can be done by wearing floatier fabrics and drapes. Don't wear anything too structured. Deep necklines work best, as they will draw the eye downwards, creating the illusion of a narrower upper half. Off-the-shoulder or wider necklines will make your top half look broader, while halter necks, one-shoulder tops or scoop necks will work really well. Fitted sleeves work well; avoid puff sleeves or any embellishment on your sleeves. When it comes to knitwear, you want to avoid adding more bulk to your top half, so go for a fine knit, rather than something chunky.

Dresses

An A-line dress is the perfect shape for an inverted triangle body shape, as it will build volume on your lower half. Dresses with pleats or patterns below the waist will also work well, as will a low V-neck dress that flares out below the bust.

Trousers and jeans

For clothing on your bottom half, you want to build up on the volume. Skinny jeans would do the opposite of that and make you look more top-heavy, so stick to looser styles.

Denim styles to try: Boyfriend-style, flares, bootcut, straight, balloon, cropped wide-leg, baggy jeans.

Jackets

Choose jackets with fluid lines, nipped-in waists and longer lengths. You can draw attention to your lower half with coats that have prints and patterns around the bottom, but avoid any details, pockets or embellishments on the top half.

Swimwear

Add volume to your bottom half to create the illusion of a balanced top and bottom by wearing prints and patterns on your lower half, or frills and ruffles. A higher leg will elongate the body, rather than draw the eye across.

Hourglass

Priyanka Chopra, Marilyn Monroe, Salma Hayek, Ashley Graham, Penelope Cruz

Your bust and hips are similar measurements, and your waist is smaller than both.

Styling tips for an hourglass shape

The key for this shape is to wear styles that accentuate your waist, but don't add any volume to your upper or lower body. Follow your natural body shape with your clothes, and don't focus too much on either the bottom or the top.

Tops

Go for tops that are fitted, tucked in and show your shape. V-necks or rounded necklines are the most flattering, while off-the-shoulder also works well, but it's best to avoid anything too voluminous. The waist is your focal point, so don't wear anything that covers it. With knitwear, go for a thinner knit, or a fine-knit cropped cardi that stops at your waist.

Dresses

You want to draw the eye towards your waist, so wear dresses that focus on this area, such as fit-and-flare styles that are tight around the waist, wrap dresses or dresses that are cut on the bias (a style that means the fabric is cut on an angle, which makes the fabric more fluid, moulding it to your body shape). Don't wear anything too boxy.

Trousers and jeans

Wide-leg, bootcut or straight-leg trousers will keep your bottom half proportionate to your top half. Make sure you stick with a mid- or high-rise (a low-rise style will cut you off at your widest point and make your legs look shorter).

Denim styles to try: Straight-leg, flare, bootcut, slim.

Jackets and coats
Fitted styles are great, nipping in at the waist. Avoid details on the shoulders or at the top, as this will set you off-balance and make you look top-heavy. Fitted blazers, wrap coats, A-line coats or princess-style coats (where the coat has a nipped-in waist and fuller skirt on the bottom) are all great shapes for an hourglass figure. Go with anything that follows the natural shape of your body.

Swimwear
Wear swimwear that has details that highlight the waist, such as a swimsuit with a belt over the waist, or a panel in a different colour in this area. For bikinis, go for a higher-leg cut, as this draws the eye upwards.

Diamond

Jennifer Hudson, Amy Schumer, Oprah Winfrey, Adele

You have a wider waist, narrow shoulders and hips with slender limbs.

Styling tips for a diamond shape
Wear clothes with shape and curves on your bottom half to balance it out with your top half. Focus on your best parts, such as bust and legs, and stick to more muted clothing around your stomach area.

Tops
You want to create a divide between your stomach and bust, so wear tops that break up this area. A well-fitting bra is imperative to lift your bust away from the stomach. A V-neck is the best neckline, as it will elongate the top half of your body. You want to make your shoulder section wider, and can do so by wearing a strapless or square neck top. You want your tops to skim over your stomach and end just below your hip line (passing the widest part of your body). Cardigans are great for

a diamond shape, as they skim the sides and draw the eye downwards, making you appear longer.

Dresses

Choose dresses that are straight then flare out towards the hem or skim the body. Wrap dresses are also ideal because they help to lift up the bust shape and create space between bust and stomach. A-line dresses and empire-line dresses can also be flattering.

Trousers and jeans

Wide-legged trousers are a perfect style for creating more curves and balance on your bottom half. Baggy trousers and cargo-style trousers also work for this body shape. Pocket details on the back will give the illusion of a more curvaceous bum. Low- or mid-rise is the best cut, as a high-rise will focus on your stomach. Stay away from a tapered cut, as this will make your top half look wider.

Denim styles to try: Bootcut, wide-leg, flare, cargo, straight-leg.

Jackets

Jackets should end just below your widest part, just on your hips, and can be a really flattering addition to your outfit. Longer-length, flowy fabrics are great as they can be elongating. It's best to avoid belted waists, as this draws the eye towards the area you don't want to focus on, but shorter jackets that are fitted at the waist can create the illusion of a waistline. A-line coats are flattering, as are straight coats. Both should be longer than your hipline.

Swimwear

You want to highlight your shoulders and legs, and keep shoulders and waist in proportion, so go for a balconette-style top with mid-rise bottoms, or a deep-V swimsuit to elongate and draw attention to shoulders and neckline.

Dressing for Your Height

Tall, petite, regular: these are terms used within the fashion industry that can play a huge role in the types of clothes you wear. Firstly, being tall or petite has absolutely nothing to do with your weight. You can be petite or tall whatever your dress size. It's about your proportions and stature, and is typically based on your height.

Within most clothing brands, 'petite' refers to someone whose height is 5 foot 3 inches (160cm) or under, and 'tall' refers to someone whose height is 5 foot 8 inches (173cm) or over. Generally, if you are between the two, then you fall into the 'regular' category. It's another reminder that women come in all shapes and sizes! There are now plenty of brands that cater towards tall and petite statures, although you'll probably find a wider selection online than in store.

No matter what category you fall into, there are some styling tricks that can create the illusion of balanced proportions.

Petite

Geri Halliwell, Nicole Richie, Octavia Spencer, Eva Longoria, Melissa McCarthy, Zoe Kravitz, Kamala Harris

'Petite' usually means a height of 5 foot 3 inches (160cm) or under, with a short torso or short legs (or both) and narrow shoulders. According to the Office of National Statistics, the average height of a woman is 5 foot 3 inches, and 50 per cent of the world's population are under 5 foot 4 inches tall.[10]

Being petite means you've probably spent your life rolling up the cuffs on your jackets, or altering the hems on your jeans. Wearing regular clothes will drown and swamp a petite frame, so you want to make sure that you wear the correct leg lengths and cuff lengths in order to avoid this. If you wear petite clothing, it will elongate your legs and arms, and won't drown your proportions. Alternatively (and if your budget allows), find a great alterations person who can make your favourite outfits maximise the potential of your frame.

TIM TOP 10: Tips for petite women

1. Vertical stripes will lengthen your torso.
2. Wear high-waisted trousers and jeans, as this will make legs appear longer.
3. Wear items that suit your frame, like structured cropped jackets.
4. Make the most of cropped tops; they'll fit full-length on you.
5. Shoes that match your skin tone will elongate your legs.
6. Avoid maxi dresses; opt for a midi instead. The maxi will drown your shape, while the midi will create space between ankles and legs, which can elongate.
7. Utilise belts to pull you in and show off your frame.
8. Maximise the French tuck – this was made for petites! Tuck in your tops only at the front or at the side, and leave the rest loose. This will instantly lengthen your legs and compliment your shape.
9. Wear shoes the same colour as your trousers. This creates the illusion of never-ending legs.
10. Go monochrome: a single colour block will vertically extend your body.

Best petite stockists

Boden, Reve The Label, John Lewis, Marks & Spencer, The Shortlist, Reformation, Me + Em, Topshop, Whistles, Reiss, Y.A.S, River Island, Nobody's Child.

Tall

Katy Perry, Serena Williams, Rihanna, Jodie Comer, Emma Thompson, Winnie Harlow, Zendaya, Adele

Items of clothing in the 'tall' category are designed to shorten a tall frame. They will all have longer hemlines and longer sleeves.

When it comes to brands catering for taller bodies, it often seems like they are at the bottom of the fashion food chain, and tall sections can be more of a challenge to find. The range for petite and regular sizes is much broader, and you have to dig deeper to find clothing that works for you if you are 5 foot 8 inches or over. Where petite folk can shorten items, taller folk can't easily add material to lengthen them.

Emily Jane Johnston (@emilyjanejohnston), one of the OG content creators (you may remember her as Fashion Foie Gras) is 5 foot 9 inches tall and an expert on dressing her tall frame. She says that the cut of most designer brands is very long: 'Too long, in fact. So if you have the money, designer prices will deliver length. But if we're talking high street, it's all about M&S, Abercrombie & Fitch and Zara.'

Speaking about how hard it was growing up as the tall kid, Emily says, 'It was so tough being thirteen and almost six feet tall. I was different, and being different as a teenager in the nineties was the last thing you wanted to be.' But as time has gone on, her opinion of her height has changed. 'As an adult, I've adored it. Sticking out, literally head and shoulders above everyone else, has been a game-changer, and one I fully embrace.'

As a tall person, you want to balance out your silhouette, and highlight certain areas, like your waistline and long limbs. Adding structure to certain areas so they become a focal point is an easy way to keep your silhouette balanced. Make the most of horizontal lines, as they will widen your frame and draw eyes across it rather than up and down.

TIM top 10: Tips for tall women

1. Cinch in your waist – it will give the illusion of a defined silhouette and break up your proportions to create balance.
2. Shop in the men's department. Oversized shirts can create volume, and the sleeves will fit well without looking shrunken.
3. Make the most of dresses. You can wear minis, midis or maxis, as long as they are the right length (going too short can highlight your long limbs, which is never a bad thing, but can make your proportions look off-balance).
4. Wear wide-legged trousers – the focus of heavier material around your ankles will balance out your height with the bottom part of your body. Just make sure they are the correct length.
5. If your torso is longer than your legs, go for shorter tops that sit on the waist. If your legs are longer than your torso, then wear longer tops that sit below your waist.
6. Use statement accessories to break up your frame. Smaller accessories can get lost and look too delicate with a taller frame.
7. Go wild with prints and patterns. You've got the space to do it, so make the most of it.
8. Break up your frame with colour. Colour blocking is a great way to separate parts of your body, like separating the top half from the bottom, and can create space within long limbs.
9. Wear well-fitting clothes. It may seem obvious, but you want to make sure your cuffs aren't too short, your shoulders aren't too pinched and your jeans are the right length. Getting this right will accentuate your frame. Show off your shape!
10. Ignore anyone who tells you not to wear heels!

Best tall stockists
Djerf Avenue, Topshop (trousers come in 34-inch and 36-inch leg lengths), Mango (they don't advertise a 'tall' range, but lots of their trousers come up long enough), Weekday (trousers come in leg lengths up to 34-inches) Asos Tall, Free People (again, they don't have a specific 'tall' section, but their dresses, skirts and jeans come in longer lengths), Abercrombie, River Island, Lucy & Yak.

Plus-Size

As a shopper and a stylist, I've seen such a positive shift in the approach to women's bodies over the years. I was once told by a very famous (male) TV executive to make sure I had the Spanx ready for a younger female artist I was styling. It made my blood boil, and is something that will stay with me for ever. (I didn't put her in the Spanx, FYI. She looked sensational without them.)

To think that people from our generation grew up surrounded by famous people saying ridiculous things like 'nothing tastes as good as skinny feels' is appalling; it must have had a huge negative impact on so many women. I'm so glad my daughter is growing up in a generation where body positivity and body inclusivity are accessible to most. Scrolling through body-positivity accounts on Instagram restores my faith in humanity.

The body-positivity movement is growing at an exponential speed, but there is still a huge way to go when it comes to fashion. Although many brands do cater for plus-sizes, the fact that some of our high-street stores stock a UK 14 as a 'large' isn't good enough.

The UK plus-size clothing market is worth £722 million, which is up 10.1 per cent compared with five years ago, and our great British high street needs to be reflecting this.

Best plus size stockists
Never Fully Dressed (up to UK size 28), New Look (up to UK 32), Monsoon (up to UK 24), Molby The Label (up to UK 24), Anthropologie Plus (up to UK 26), Asos Curve (UK 18–30)

TV presenter, DJ and body-positivity advocate Ashley James says that her style has evolved with her confidence. 'Society tells us we are happiest when at our smallest, but for me the opposite is true. When I allowed my body to just be and I started nurturing it with movement and eating intuitively, I found I thought less about food and my weight. Now I don't stress about having rolls when I sit down, or an overhang on my hips on my jeans – because I've stopped trying to squeeze into clothes that don't fit. Why do we get so caught up on a number stitched onto clothing anyway?' Ashley now uses various styling tips to help her feel her best in clothes. 'I've discovered more flattering shapes and actually prefer looser fitting clothing. I guess I've stopped dressing for the patriarchy, even though I did so subconsciously. I've realised that being the smallest most shrunken version of yourself usually doesn't equate to happiness and confidence.'

Ashley has a large bust and has learnt over the years how to dress her own shape.

'There's so much stigma around a big bust, and a presumption that you're attention seeking or wanting male attention (even when the opposite is true). I used to think I had to wear tight-fitting clothing so you could see my shape and so I didn't look bigger. Now I realise that there's no harm in looking bigger first and foremost. But also, there are ways to dress cool, but still show your figure. High-waist jeans. Wearing belts! Tucking baggy jumpers into waist belts. Showing off ankles by doing a skinny tuck fold. Showing off my wrists by wearing arm garters. Sizing up with shirts, but also ensuring things are well fitted under the arms. There are so many tips and tricks!'

Modest Dressing

Modest dressing refers to dressing in a way that shows less skin and is less revealing. People do this for a number of reasons, including religious reasons or personal preference. Modest dressing can draw attention towards your inner personality, rather than your physical features.

One of the UK's top beauty editors, Jessica Diner, started dressing modestly when she converted to Judaism more than a decade ago, as a way of affirming her faith. Jessica says that dressing modestly is now part of her, in the same way that her religion is part of her. When discussing what dressing modestly means to her, Jessica says, 'While at this point it's pretty much second nature, looking in my wardrobe and seeing all my dresses hanging up every morning is a lovely reminder of [making] a concerted effort to dress in a way that is purposeful and has meaning. It elevates an everyday ritual.'

She says that dressing modestly has never been easier. 'You just have to autotune your radar. When I go into any shop app, I filter by dress or skirt length, select "midi or maxi", and there will always be ample choice. I'm the same in a physical store, too. I just scan the rails for the longer lengths and go straight to peruse those items. There is the common misconception that to dress modestly means eschewing what is "fashionable" or "cool", but the reality is, it's all in how you wear it and how you carry yourself in tandem.'

■ ■ ■

Whether you fit into a tall or petite category, have an hourglass shape or are more diamond-shaped (or something in the middle), please remember that at different stages in our lives, society will try to tell us that one is better than another – but this is irrelevant. And although ignoring a narrative like this is much easier said than done, I hope that this chapter will have helped you gain some confidence in whatever body shape you are. If you still find it hard to visualise styling ideas, then look up the ladies who have been mentioned as having a similar body shape to yours and take some inspiration from them and their outfits. You can also look on Pinterest or the Like To Know It app (LTK), as both are an easy way to find and follow people of the same shape or size who may inspire you with their outfits.

- 8 -

how to build outfits

Once you've cleared out and organised your wardrobe, worked out your personal style, and defined your body shape, you will want to start building outfits. By this point, you should have your wardrobe set up so you can quickly and easily build outfits in a way that suits you best. Obviously, this will all depend on your own personal style, but how you combine these pieces of clothing together is what makes the outfit complete and wearable. This chapter shares how to put together all the pieces in your wardrobe to create outfits.

Where to Start

Basics: tops and bottoms

It can be hard to work out where to start, but the easiest thing to do is to pull out one top you love. If you struggle to choose, then go for something you haven't worn in a while. Next, you want to find bottoms that work with the top.

As you make these choices, think about:

- Where are you going?
- How do you want to feel (smart/casual/powerful/comfortable, etc)?

- What is the weather like?
- Does the colour of the top match the bottoms?
- If the top and/or bottoms have a print or pattern, do they work well together?
- Do the shapes work well together? For example, if the top is fitted, it's more flattering to wear looser bottoms, and vice versa.

Layers

Next up, do you need layers? Would a cardigan or knitwear work, or would a leather jacket work better with your personal style? Does the outfit need more structure?

Shoes

Once you've layered up, you can think about shoes. What do the proportions of the outfit look like together? If the focus of the outfit is on the top, do you need to balance out the bottom a bit by adding a chunkier shoe, or a shoe in a darker colour? If the outfit is quite bottom-heavy, then go for a more delicate, subtle shoe.

Accessories

Finally, add some accessories: belts, bags and jewellery. You can use jewellery to add more elements of your personal style, or a statement bag to make the outfit feel more powerful. A belt can cinch it at the right place to create a flattering silhouette.

Check out how your outfit looks and feels. If you feel like it isn't working, then switch out one of your basic items for something totally different; this usually does the trick.

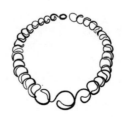

Colour

Colour can play a huge role in how the outfit comes together, and it can help to make an outfit look more expensive than it is. The colours you wear can also have a huge impact on your mood. Within the fashion industry, we often talk about dopamine dressing, and there has been a fair amount of research into proving this as a valid theory. Dopamine is a neurotransmitter (a chemical messenger in the body), and it plays a role in the brain's reward system. There isn't any evidence yet that shows putting on a certain colour will give us a mood boost, but there is some evidence showing that the brain responds in a certain way when it sees a certain colour. It all comes back to the idea that we should dress for how we want to feel, rather than dressing for how we *do* feel in that moment. One study showed that football teams wearing red performed significantly better than any other team over a period of fifty-five years (note to self: tell my husband to switch from Spurs and support a team that wear red!).[11]

I've never been a fan of colour consultations (where someone tells you which colours suit you best), and I don't think it's a wise way to spend your money. Yes, sure, we all have colours that make us look and feel great, and can complement our hair or eyes, but it's not a one-size-fits-all kind of thing. Have you ever heard that blondes shouldn't wear yellow? Just look at Holly Willoughby and Margot Robbie, both of whom epitomise beauty and joy when they wear sunny shades.

Zeena Shah, author, stylist, designer and queen of dopamine dressing, says: 'Reds are energising, whereas cooler, more pastel shades bring calmness. If you're new to wearing colour, I always suggest starting small. Add a colourful handbag, accessory or pair of socks, or paint your nails in a bright shade, and you'll instantly notice the difference to your mood.'

Using colour can also be a quick way to get some inspiration for pulling things together when you aren't sure of what to wear. Just choose two colours – check the colour wheel for inspiration, and choose two opposite colours if you are feeling bold – then sift through your wardrobe and see what you can find that works together. Colour blocking in particular is a great way to build outfits.

Here are a few colour combinations that work well together without clashing.

- lilac and orange
- blue and green
- red and pink (my personal favourite!)
- purple and orange
- pink and blue
- orange and yellow
- purple and pink
- red and green
- purple and yellow
- brown and cream
- black and brown
- red and brown
- navy and black (yes, really – it looks so chic!)

If colour blocking isn't your thing, then another way to build an outfit quickly is to go monochrome. Monochrome means wearing one colour from head to toe, or wearing black and white. If you go for one colour head to toe, then there are some easy ways to break up the look, and make it look styled and well pulled together with minimal effort involved.

TIM top 10: Tips for wearing monochrome looks

1. Add accessories to break it up so the look isn't so intense.
2. Keep it casual – throw on some trainers, or add a leather jacket over bold colours.
3. Take a broader approach to your monochromatic look – if blue is the chosen colour, add denim. If grey is the chosen colour, add silver. If yellow is the chosen colour, add gold.
4. Combine textures and prints – don't be afraid to wear two different pink prints together. Keep one print larger (bold stripes) and one smaller (a ditzy floral.) Using different textures (like silks with fur, for example) can also create a contrast within the outfit.
5. Wear muted tones. If going for a bold colour from head to toe doesn't feel comfortable or doesn't fit in with your personal style, then try a more muted colour palette with browns, or creams, greys or blacks.
6. Wear basics – you don't need to go overboard. If a very dressed-up monochromatic look feels like too much for you, then just try it out with grey joggers and a grey T-shirt, or blue jeans with a blue top.
7. Add structure. If it all feels a bit out of sync, then pull in the look with sharp shoulders or tailored trousers.
8. Pinterest is a great source of colour inspiration for outfit building. You can search for your base item in a colour; for example, 'grey T-shirt outfit styling' and it will bring up lots of visual options.
9. If in doubt, then just add one small detail in a different colour, like a belt or bag, or even add brightly coloured socks to black jeans and loafers.
10. If it doesn't feel like 'you', then add some pieces from your capsule wardrobe to tone it down, like your favourite jeans, or a leather jacket or denim shirt. This is an easy way to start playing with colour.

Wearing Clothes vs Styling Clothes

We all want to look more like we've put thought and effort into what we wear – ideally without actually *having* to put in any thought or effort! People often say that the French look effortlessly chic, but this is because they 'style' their outfits, rather than just *wearing* them. This can sound quite intense or like hard work, but in reality there are many tiny tweaks you can make to your outfits to make them look more styled, and these little things will gradually become habits that you do without thinking. It's all about creating your new norm; once this is created, it will become second nature, and it won't take you any extra time or effort to include these new rituals in your morning routine before you dash out the door.

TIM top 10: Simple styling tricks

Here are ten of my favourite easy tricks for when you want your outfit to look more styled, but you've only had five hours of sleep and now have five minutes to get ready. Each tip is simple, easy to do and doesn't take a lot of time once you've done it once or twice, and they will all pull an outfit together when you are running out the house.

1. **Elongate your legs:** High-waisted jeans or trousers will instantly make your legs look longer. Essentially, changing from a low-rise style to either mid- or high-rise can add inches to your legs.

2. **Balance proportions:** Keeping your proportions aligned can help with the overall aesthetic of an outfit. If you are top-heavy (busty with broad shoulders), then use something to draw the eye downwards and elongate, such as a blazer with long, thin lapels, or a long necklace. If you are bottom-heavy and smaller on top, keep your bottom half plain, and add the prints and details to your top half.

3. **Wear the right length:** Wearing jeans that are too long and crinkle around your ankles will make your legs look shorter, but jeans that are too short will cut you off at the wrong point, which can *also* make your legs look shorter! Many brands offer a range of leg lengths, so make sure you go for the right one.

4. **Roll your cuffs:** When wearing a blazer or shirt, if you simply roll up your cuffs so you can see some wrist, it can make such a difference to the overall look of an outfit. It makes it look more styled, and can also help balance your proportions, as it creates space in the outfit around your arms and helps it look effortless and relaxed.

5. **Add jewellery:** If in doubt, add jewels. If you are rushing to get ready, or don't have the time or inspiration to plan an outfit, then just wear jeans and a T-shirt, but add jewellery. It instantly elevates your look, makes it look like you've made more effort

than was required, and can make the most basic of outfits look styled.

6. **Wear a belt:** It may sound basic, but adding a belt can do so much to an outfit. It can pull a look together, it can create more definition within your shape, and it can make an outfit look more expensive and chic. It can even lengthen your legs!

7. **Dress for how you want to feel:** Don't dress for your current mood. Clothes can be so powerful. Even if you are working from home, or just doing some errands, if you want to feel good, then put on a proper outfit (as opposed to loungewear). Add a lip, a blazer or a pretty blouse. It can have a huge impact.

8. **Textures can make it interesting:** Wearing different textures together can elevate a look. Think about how everything feels. Mix leathers with denim, and knits with silks.

9. **Add tailoring:** Any structure added to an outfit will make you feel like you are physically pulled together. A tailored blazer is one of the most useful items you can own, and will elevate jeans and a T-shirt, leggings and an oversized jumper with boots, or a simple midi dress.

10. **Choose one statement piece:** When I'm in a hurry, I wear a monochromatic look, and then choose one item to stand out, whether it's a statement bag, oversized earrings or a bold top. This way, the look stays polished without being fussy.

■ ■ ■

Stick a bookmark in this chapter and if you are ever in a fashion tizz, unsure of what to wear and needing to get out of the door stat, then you can refer back to it. Hopefully it will inspire you with your outfit choice. Even with minimal time and effort, a few simple hacks will leave you feeling great.

- 9 -

the future of fashion

I grew up in a household of vintage and antique items, and remember watching my mum get such a kick out of finding something old and restoring it into something valuable and new. It's been ingrained in me from a young age that buying vintage is a more sensible and sustainable choice. However, that doesn't mean that I don't get excited about finding a new outfit, or that I haven't done my fair share of fast-fashion shopping.

I was part of the generation when ASOS was known as 'AsSeenOnScreen', where you'd have a new outfit for every occasion, and going to 'Big Topshop' at Oxford Circus was like a weekend sport. But I always had eBay as my side hustle! I saved for the deposit on my first flat by selling clothes online. I'd spy a pair of coveted shoes on sale in a store, buy them and put them on eBay. Or I'd find 'the' dress Kate Moss had worn, list it and stay up late to watch the bidding war commence.

As I've got older and had children, I've realised more and more the impact that our fashion choices have, and although it's impossible to be perfect, I've made a conscious decision to lead a more eco-friendly lifestyle as much as possible. This has meant cutting back hugely on buying new, checking the labels to make sure I only buy natural fabrics and making wiser choices when it comes to my wardrobe.

Below are some tips that can help you make more sustainable fashion choices – and, surprisingly, they aren't as time-consuming, difficult or expensive as you may think. There are really simple, day-to-day things that you can do that can make a huge difference to our planet.

TIM top 10: Simple fashion for a more sustainable future

1. **Wash your clothing less:** 700,000 microfibres (tiny pieces of plastic) can detach in one single wash and ultimately make their way to our oceans and lakes, so think twice before you put a load in the machine.

2. **Use fabric refresher sprays:** My favourite is byMATTER's Another Day spray, as it has no harsh chemicals, eliminates odours and gets rid of harmful bacteria.

3. **Wear natural (ideally organic) fabrics rather than synthetic:** I discuss this in more detail opposite.

4. **Avoid fast fashion:** This is easier said than done, of course, mainly because our choices come down to budget. But if your budget allows, then shop small, ethical brands that are transparent with their journey from design to finished garment so you can see how eco-friendly they are.

5. **Go for quality over quantity:** If you must buy new, then make sure it's something that will last. Check the craftsmanship in zips and seams, and make sure it's durable. It will save you money in the long run, and is of course better for the planet.

6. **Educate yourself:** There is so much easily accessible information out there. One of my favourite documentaries is Amy Powney's *Fashion Reimagined*. It follows her journey as she creates a fully sustainable collection with her fashion label Mother of Pearl. It is so insightful, not only for people who work in fashion, but for literally anyone and everyone who wears clothes (watch it on Sky Documentaries or Now TV).

7. **Don't throw any clothing in the bin:** If it's still wearable, then share it with friends, give it to a neighbour, donate it to charity or sell it on a resale site. If it's not wearable, then find your local textile recycling point. The clothing can then be recycled and turned into something new. Recyclenow.com is a great source for working out where to recycle. You can search by item (it's not

only restricted to clothing) and enter your postcode, and it will show the nearest location to you for the relevant item. If it gets thrown in the bin, it will end up in landfill.

8. **Rent your wardrobe:** Gone are the days when we needed to have something new for a night out. There is absolutely no need to ever buy something new for a special occasion. You can rent any outfit, from wedding dresses to a powerful suit for an interview.

9. **Buy second-hand:** We are inundated with brands selling second-hand or pre-loved clothes these days, with everything on offer from high-street to high-end. Check out eBay, Vinted, Vestiaire Collective, FarFetch and Selfridges for pre-loved gems. More on this starting on page 168.

10. **Don't buy it right away:** It's so rare that we actually *need* to buy clothes, so make sure you second-guess yourself. Sleep on it, ask yourself how often you would wear it, ask yourself if you'd benefit from owning it, or if you just want it because of the kick you get from buying something.

The Fabric Guide

There are two main types of fabrics, natural and synthetic. There can be pros and cons to both, but in a world where living as sustainably as possible is more important than ever, going for natural fabrics can have a huge positive impact on our planet. So, where possible, avoid synthetics.

Natural fabrics

Natural fabrics are plant, animal or mineral derived. They are biodegradable, meaning that ultimately, at the end of their life, they will be broken down naturally by other living things or bacteria. Natural fibres are also comfortable to wear, as they are breathable and excellent at absorbing moisture, which makes it less likely that you will get sweaty when wearing them. They are also naturally hypo-allergenic, and they have antibacterial properties within the fabrics, so if you tend to suffer from rashes/allergies/eczema or any skin conditions then they won't cause a reaction.

Most common natural fabrics: Cotton, silk, linen, wool, mohair, jute, cashmere

Synthetic fabrics

Synthetic fabrics are man-made, with chemicals used in the fibre-making process. They can take hundreds of years to decompose (if they ever do). Synthetics are much cheaper to source, use and buy, which is why they are so commonly found on the high street. Although they take so long to decompose fully, most synthetics break down quickly, so tiny plastic particles (known as microfibres) shed off as you wear them and wash them. These end up in our wastewater, and as they are so small, they pass through filtration systems and end up in rivers and oceans. The microplastics from our clothing result in a whopping 34.8 per cent of global microplastic pollution.

Most common synthetic fabrics: Polyester, nylon, acrylic, fleece, spandex

In short, go for natural fabrics where you can. They are good for your wardrobe (because of the longevity of your clothing) and even better for the planet.

The Care Guide

The end goal when it comes to your wardrobe is to minimise buying new, and to own clothes that last. There are plenty of things you can do to make sure they endure the test of time. If you wear them well, wash them well and store them well, you can help the longevity of your favourite pieces. This involves really getting to know your clothes, checking the labels before washing them and looking after them as best you can. Here is some advice on how to do so.

TIM top 10: How to treat your clothes with care

1. **Wash by colour:** This sounds obvious, and I know it is so tempting to bung them all in at once, but separating clothes into colours before you wash will help with longevity. Make a pile of whites, a pile of pastels, a pile of bold colours and a pile of darks. This prevents any dye transfers and fading.

2. **Read the care labels:** They are there for a reason, and you might be surprised at what the instructions are. We'll look at this in more detail on page 165.

3. **Soak your swimwear:** Let your swimwear soak in cold water, ideally for thirty minutes, after every single wear. Soaking it removes most of the bacteria, body oils and chlorine that can damage the fabric and cause colours to fade, elasticity to loosen and fibres to break down. The cold water alone is a good start, and will help lengthen the lifespan of your swimwear, but ideally you also want to use a mild detergent (or, if you don't have one, a little dollop of shampoo or some distilled white vinegar). Squeeze out the excess water (never wring out swimwear) then lay it flat to dry out of direct sunlight, as this will cause colours to fade. I learned this the hard way when I was lazy with my Barbie-pink Hunza G. Also, don't wear your best swimwear in a hot tub – the

chemicals and heat are a bad combination, and will only encourage loss of colour and shape quicker than anywhere else.

4. **Treat stains immediately:** The longer you leave them, the harder they will be to remove, because they settle into the fabric. Blot stains, don't rub, and always treat the stain before putting it into the washing machine. If you bung it in without treating it, the stain will be impossible to remove once it's washed.

5. **Keep your jewellery clean:** You don't need anything fancy: an old toothbrush and a dab of fairy liquid will usually do the job to make jewels and gems more sparkly. This works particularly well on diamonds.

6. **Cold washes do just as good a job as hot:** Not doing a hot wash is a hard habit to crack, and it also doesn't sound like it should make sense, but washing at 30°C not only saves energy, it also helps keep your clothes vibrant in colour and reduces shrinkage.

7. **Don't use wire hangers:** They will ruin the shape of your clothes. Stick to velvet with soft edges.

8. **Don't be afraid of mending:** Mending clothes isn't as big a job as you may think it is. A strap breaking on a dress isn't a reason to buy a new one. Your local tailor, dry-cleaner or alterations shop will most likely be able to fix something for a really reasonable price – or you can have a go yourself with a needle and thread. It's never as hard as it seems. Check out specialist repair company @the.seam.uk on Instagram for inspo on how to fix items, from moth holes to ripped knees.

9. **Check if something is well made before purchasing:** Look for strong zips (YKK are usually the strongest), and check there are no loose threads. Pull the fabric to see if it goes back to its original shape, and look at the patterns to see if they match up at the seams.

10. **Apply perfume, hairsprays and deodorants before you get dressed and give them a moment to dry:** They all contain chemicals, and the build-up of these chemicals can damage and stain clothing.

Know your care labels

There is a care label on every single item of clothing you buy, and each one contains information and instructions on how to look after your clothes correctly. It's always worth following what the label says, as this will help with the longevity of the item. The glossary has a guide to each symbol.

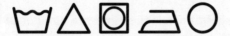

How to keep your whites white

If you find your whites getting a bit grey or yellow, then add some baking soda to the washing cycle.

Try to let perfume and deodorant dry properly before putting on white clothing, and apply make-up afterwards. Alternatively, if make-up has gone on first, then pop a silk scarf over your face and pull the T-shirt down over it so you don't get any make-up stains on the T-shirt.

Some SPFs (and if you've read Sam's chapters, you should know you must be wearing SPF 365 days a year!) can cause yellow stains around the neckline of T-shirts. Some sun creams contain avobenzone, and this ingredient, combined with anything containing iron (like water, e.g. from the swimming pool or the sea), can create a rust stain. So it isn't technically an SPF stain that you'd use a normal fabric stain remover to tackle; it's a rust stain, and that means you need something that specifically removes rust.

Similarly, if you find the armpits on your white T-shirts get stained yellow, this can be because of a chemical reaction with your sweat and the aluminium in your deodorant. Switch to a natural deodorant, or again, you can use a fabric rust remover (on the clothes, not on your armpits!).

I use Dr Beckman's Stain Expert: Rust & Deodorant. Don't try bleach – rust is the one stain that bleach won't work on. Because of the oxidising agent in bleach, it will just cause it to rust even more, and the stain will go pink. If you'd prefer something more natural, then wet the stain, squeeze some lemon juice over it, then pour table salt over the whole stain and leave it overnight. The next day, brush off the salt and then wash the top as normal, and the stain should come out.

Remove the bobbles

Bobbling (or pilling) happens when parts of a material become loose. Instead of just falling off, they get knotted up within the fabric and form a cluster of fabric or balls. This process is usually caused by friction on the fabric, so it's more likely to happen once the piece of clothing has been in the washing machine (where it will have rubbed up against other clothes), or if it's been squashed onto a shelf. Bobbling may also occur under your sleeves as a result of you moving your arms back and forth, or on the side of your coat thanks to your bag rubbing against it. Even the most expensive knitwear can bobble, so don't think that splashing out on a cute jumper from a luxury brand will make any difference. That said, cheaper fabrics and synthetic fabrics *will* be more likely to break and snap faster, as they are more poorly made. Luckily, there are a few things you can do to prevent the bobbling, or at least minimise it.

Wash items alone

Ideally, do this by hand. It's a waste of water and not good for the environment to wash just one item in a washing machine. Fill the sink with tepid water, add a handwash detergent (my favourite is Ecover's Wool & Silk Laundry Detergent), then turn the garment inside out and immerse fully in the sink. Leave to sit for ten minutes. Don't panic if the colour of the water changes; this will only be excess dye and won't affect the overall colour of the garment. Rinse it thoroughly (you can use a colander for this if it's easier), then squeeze out the water with both hands by squashing the garment from top to bottom. Never, ever wring it – this can cause it to lose its shape. Then lay it flat, either on a drying rack, or on a towel, as this can absorb the excess water. You can roll up the towel with the garment inside it (like a tortilla wrap) if you want it to dry faster. This will suck up more water. Then lay it flat on a dry towel to dry fully while keeping its shape. If you have a big enough sink, then you can wash multiples together, but ideally you should wash garments of the same colour at the same time.

Use a short delicates cycle

Handwashing is great if you have the time (and is actually much quicker than you'd think) but if you do need to use the machine, it's best to do a quick wash so that the clothing isn't spun round and round, over and over. Always turn delicate garments inside out for a bit of extra protection, and opt for a liquid detergent rather than powder. The liquid will dissolve immediately, while the powder has to dissolve throughout the wash.

Don't use the tumble-dryer

This is probably the thing that will cause the most bobbling. The friction from the clothes spinning, combined with the heat, can cause the fibres in your jumpers to tear, so avoid this at all costs. As explained above, air-drying while laid flat will help your clothes to keep their shape.

Use fabric shavers or debobbling combs

Electric fabric shavers are really time-efficient, but you must use them with care. Going over and over one area of bobbling can weaken the rest of the fabric, and may even cause a hole. I've debobbled for years and years, and my tool of choice would always be a comb. It can take a while, but settle down on the couch with your favourite trashy TV show (my debobbling TV show is *Below Deck*, in case you were wondering!) and work your way around the top in a methodical manner so you don't miss any patches. It's pretty therapeutic. You could also use Velcro or duct tape to save you buying a new 'tool'.

Shop wisely

Merino wool is least likely to bobble because it's so tightly woven together and is so strong. So if bobbling really bothers you, then go for merino wool. Uniqlo has a great selection of merino. And don't forget to check the men's department – oversized knits always look chic with denim.

Renting, Buying and Sourcing Second-Hand Clothes

As I mentioned earlier, I've been buying and selling on eBay since early 2000, and I still do it to this day. I've recently also jumped on to the Vinted bandwagon and managed to sell off quite a few bits and pieces from my wardrobe that I no longer wear, as well as some clothes my kids have grown out of.

Throughout my years of buying and selling, I've picked up a few tips.

TIM top 10: Tips for buying on re-sell sites

1. Be as descriptive as possible in your search box so you can narrow down the search. Search for the specific brand, size and condition you're looking for.
2. Use the filters to make it easier to find what you're after.
3. Check the location of the item so you don't get caught out and have to pay extra customs fees.
4. Triple-check the condition so you don't miss anything. You can also ask for extra pictures, which will help you to visually confirm the condition.
5. Ask the seller as many questions as you like. They want to sell the item, so will be happy to answer.

6. Check if there is a returns policy.

7. Try typing in some common misspellings, as sometimes people make a mistake when writing their listings. For example, search for 'Channel' – I once won a pair of genuine Chanel sunglasses for £15, as the seller had made this error.

8. If you are looking for designer items, then make sure it is stated in the description that the item is 100 per cent authentic. If this isn't made clear, then send the seller a message to check.

9. Check the seller's previous feedback. If the majority of it is positive, you can feel confident that they are a trustworthy seller.

10. If you're looking at a luxury-brand item, then ask the seller for a copy or photo of the receipt. If they bought it in a store, they should have proof.

The genuine article

If you are specifically looking for a designer item, then there are a few things worth checking. If the item is genuine, the stitching will be impeccable and the prints or patterns will match up at the seams. Ask where the item was made, or ask for a picture of the label that states where it was made, then do your research. For example, from a quick Google search, you can see that Louis Vuitton bags are made in France, Spain, Italy and America. So if the bag or the listing states it was made in China, then it's a fake.

Counterfeit items are illegal and should not be sold on any re-sale site. Most of the popular sites, like Vinted, eBay and Vestiaire, have a team dedicated to monitoring the fakes, but some still slip through. If you buy something and it turns out to be fake, then don't panic. You should be entitled to a full refund; just make sure you report it as soon as possible.

TIM top 10: Tips for selling on re-sale sites

1. The more open and descriptive you are when selling, the more likely it is that your item will go for a good price.
2. Provide as many clear photos as possible on a clean background. Clothing looks best if it's hung on a hanger, or laid flat on a clean surface.
3. There is no point hiding a hole or stain, as you'll only end up having to refund the buyer.
4. Use a clear title with as many 'searchable' words as possible. Think about what you'd type in if you were searching for this item, for example: 'Black Topshop knitted jumper, size UK 12, brand new.' This way, anyone who searches for any of those words – such as 'black jumper', 'Topshop jumper' or 'size 12 jumper '– will see your item.
5. Explain how the seller has to pay (e.g. PayPal, cash on collection, etc.).
6. State in the description whether you accept returns (it's usually easier not to!).
7. State in the description if you are selling other items, as the buyer can then look through the rest of the clothes you have listed.
8. Add the size, colours and fabrics to the description.
9. If you have a bunch of similar items in the same size, you can sell them as a 'job lot' or a 'bundle', which means you sell them all together. It's a great way to shift a pile of clothes that you don't wear and make some money from them.
10. Sell on the right website. I tend to stick to eBay for luxury-brand items, as they have a great audience for that. I post my high-street clothes on Vinted, because the audience seems a bit younger and more bargain-savvy. If you've got teenagers' clothes to shift, then Depop is the best place for it, as it has a huge Gen Z audience. Vestiaire is great if you want them to authenticate

and sell the item for you, but it's worth noting that they take a 25 per cent commission. If you are time-poor, then Reluxe can carry out the entire process for you, including collecting it from your home. They take around a 35 per cent commission, depending on what the item is.

TIM top 10: Second-hand and slow fashion stores

If you don't want to trawl through eBay or scroll through pages of Vinted, then there are plenty of second-hand brands out there, as well as small businesses who sell new clothing but consider the process and resources of the clothing being made. The clothing is never trend-led, will last years longer than fast fashion ever would, and is made from only natural, recycled or sustainable fabrics. The following list is from my little black book – don't share them with anyone else, okay?!

1. **Susan Caplan:** First up, my all-time favourite vintage jewellery brand – not *just* because it's my mum's brand, but mainly because she is such a brilliant buyer with a sharp eye. All the pieces she buys are unique, with a story to tell, and will last a lifetime.
2. **The Hosta:** My go-to brand for pre-loved bags. It's worth following on Instagram, as owner Danni shares her new-in bags on there first, and the good ones get snapped up quickly.
3. **Seventy & Mochi:** A female-led brand founded in 2020 and a personal favourite of mine. They specialise in denim, with a twist. Think cute blouses, boiler suits and brilliant-fitting jeans.
4. **Beyond Nine:** My ultimate go-to brand for comfy, wearable, everyday slouchy clothing, including oversized tracksuits, comfy boilersuits and jumpsuits. The brand launched with the idea of selling clothes that would see you from pre-pregnancy, through pregnancy and beyond, with the ethos that even though your body changes, your clothes don't have to. The pieces have drawstrings or poppers so you can expand or tighten waistlines.

5. **Reluxe:** If you are looking for something a bit more niche, then Reluxe is the place for you. It's a fairly new website selling second-hand designer items. Each item states the condition and the photography is really clear, so you can have a thorough check of the items you love.

6. **Ninety Percent:** If you need to build up on your basics collection then Ninety Percent is where you should look. Simple, classic, layering pieces that are made from responsible vegan materials, built to last. Ninety per cent of their profits get shared out – 80 per cent to charitable causes and 10 per cent to the people who create the collections.

7. **Damson Madder:** A fairly new brand which started in 2020, born out of a need for slower, more considered and more responsible fashion. Bold prints and patterns on fashion-forward pieces, like leopard print gilets and floral dresses, with a size range from UK 6–20.

8. **People Tree:** This brand was one of my first freelance styling clients about ten years ago. They are among the pioneers of ethical fashion, first launching in 1991 and still going strong more than thirty years later. The brand features simple day-to-day clothing, made to the highest ethical standards.

9. **Charity shops:** One of my favourite weekend activities is mooching in a charity shop. Go to an affluent area and have a browse through their charity-shop offerings. This is where the wealthier people who live in the area will donate their clothes, so you could snap up a bargain. I've often spotted Louis Vuitton and Mui Mui in Oxfam on Marylebone High Street in London.

10. **Car boot sales:** Another great place to snap up a good deal. I once got some leopard-print Moschino trousers for £7. Yes, you have to sift through a fair amount of stuff to find what you are looking for, but there are always some gems hiding in there. Have a google for car boot sales if you are going on a staycay they are usually better when they aren't near big cities.

Fashion rentals

As we've all become more aware of the impact that the fashion industry has on the environment, we're all (finally!) realising that we don't need to buy something new for every special occasion we attend (and it actually makes me feel a bit sick that we all used to do this!). You can still get the kick out of wearing something new, though – just rent an outfit. We already rent cars, homes, parking spaces, tools and sports equipment, so it's surprising it's taken so long for us to catch on to renting our wardrobes too.

American company Rent the Runway were the first brand to try this out, way back in 2009. They initially launched online, gradually expanding to include accessories and plus-size clothing before opening their first standalone store in New York City in 2014 – way ahead of their time! The company was valued at $1 billion in 2019, so they were obviously doing something right!

Renting is a great way to try out something you wouldn't normally go for, and is also a brilliant option if you need an outfit for a special occasion. You can even rent a wedding dress. There has recently been a huge increase in the number of stores and brands you can rent from, with many high-street department stores now offering the option of renting new-in clothes within their stores.

You can even make extra cash by renting out your own wardrobe. Companies like Hurr offer this service, which runs in a similar way to Airbnb. You can share your wardrobe, chat with the person who wants to rent from you, and then you have a certain time period in which you can accept or decline the rental offer. Hurr has a £150 minimum price point, which they have in place in order to cut out fast-fashion brands, but this doesn't mean they only hold very high-end brands. There are so many mid-level brands that will last the test of time, like Ganni, Rixo & Rotate, and many other new and emerging brands you may not have heard of yet. As an added plus, if you have clothes you no longer wear, then Hurr can donate them to Traid on your behalf so they don't end up in landfill.

TIM TOP 10: Fashion rental companies

1. **Hurr:** Available online, or in store in Selfridges. You can hire – and rent out – items ranging from high-end high-street pieces to luxury brands.
2. **By Rotation:** This was the first UK rental service to have an app. You can rent out your own wardrobe on it and hire items from others. You also have the option to buy a piece you've previously rented if you love it.
3. **Cocoon Club:** A bag-only rental site that runs on a subscription basis.
4. **John Lewis:** They've recently launched their own rental service, and you can rent brands from Whistles to Marchesa.
5. **For The Creators:** It always seemed absurd that people would buy maternity items when they fall pregnant, and only wear them for a year at the most. For The Creators rents items for during pregnancy and your first trimester.
6. **Cloan:** Cloan works slightly differently to other rental sites, as every item is owned by them, so you're not renting out someone else's wardrobe. Each item is professionally cleaned and sent out directly from Cloan.
7. **Hirestreet:** A high-street rental site that has simple filters to help you refine your selection to save time (and avoid scrolling).
8. **Susan Caplan:** Looking for some jewellery to go with an evening dress, but don't have any more occasions to wear it for? Susan Caplan, the globally renowned vintage jewellery brand that stocks beautiful jewels is planning to offer jewels for hire from £10 up to £5,000 in 2024. I've already told you that this is my mum's brand, but in all honesty, I'd be just as obsessed if she wasn't my mum!
9. **My Wardrobe HQ:** The go-to place for luxury-brand rentals. They also offer a resale service in case you fall in love with one of the pieces you rent.
10. **Selfridges:** They offer their own rental platform as part of their Project Earth initiative. You can rent out from a huge array of the designers and brands that they stock.

I hope this chapter has encouraged you to think twice before you buy something new. If you do find yourself in need of a particular item, I hope the resources I've shared will help you look for different places to shop or even rent. It is becoming increasingly simple to keep fashion circular, and while it's so easy to just stick with what we know (usually because we are time-poor, or out of convenience – hello, I'm totally the same!), we are learning that by shopping second-hand, renting clothes or selling our own unwanted items, we can help with the awful environmental impact the fashion industry has on the planet. Plus, you can save – or even make – some money by doing so!

■ ■ ■

And so we've come to the end of the fashion section of this book. I hope more than anything that this has helped you gain some sort of confidence in putting outfits together, clearing out what you don't need and investing in what you *do* need. I hope you've learned a few things along the way about how important it is for our planet that we make wise fashion choices. It's not about going the whole hog, because this isn't always realistic – and I'd be lying if I said I didn't ever enjoy a quick scroll-and-add-to-basket on a fast-fashion website. But my shopping habits have changed hugely over the years, and if we all make the effort to make small changes and form new habits, it will make a huge difference.

Remember: if you are having a bad day, feeling a bit 'meh' and don't know what to wear, put on head-to-toe black, layer on your jewellery and a leather jacket, and I guarantee you will feel more confident and powerful than you did when you first woke up. If that doesn't work, then pick an outfit that's based on how you *want* to feel, not how you feel in that moment. And if all else fails, wear whatever the heck you want and what makes you feel wonderful right now. There is no wrong answer when it comes to fashion.

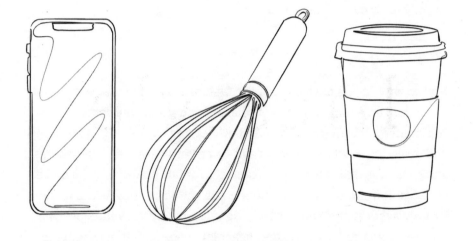

- part three -

lifestyle

...

We have decades of professional expertise in the fashion and beauty industries, and we can offer you skincare tips and styling tricks until the cows come home, but something else has happened over the last ten years or so. We've somehow become accidental authorities on the three Hs: Holidays, Home hacks and – our mums can't actually believe it – Hosting grown-up dinner parties. Somewhere amongst the hectic pace of working life, we've dragged ourselves up from being twenty-somethings who would burn an oven pizza (well, Gemma sometimes still burns pizza), couldn't for the life of them find a clean pair of socks, and thought nothing of planning a last-minute girls' trip to NYC even when the bank balance said not to, to somehow becoming thirty-somethings who are able to cater a dinner party for ten, smooth creases out of a shirt in seconds, and act as oracles on which time zones are best to travel to for optimum sunshine each month of the year. And although it might not be the glam kind of content our Insta feed shows, it's become part of our lives that we really enjoy, and so we wanted to share these things with you. This is the kind of information everyone needs to know in order to run a streamlined life: the knowledge that will help you to wing it when you feel like you are dropping all the balls.

Gemma & Sam x

- 10 -

the TIM method at home

The Invisible Load

We could talk about 'the invisible load' for hours. The invisible load is the behind-the-scenes work that goes into running a house as a modern-day woman. It can be logistical, physical, emotional or mental. This hidden work is hard to measure *precisely* because it's hidden. It's performed internally: adding toilet roll to the online shop; making sure the laundry makes it out of the machine; remembering to buy a birthday present for your friend's fortieth.

There's enough here to require a book all of its own, and we are sure there are many of them out there, but when you feel like you are drowning, we're not sure there's really enough brain space to read a whole book about it. While we can't ease your load, we do think there is power in knowing you're not alone.

The saying 'tidy house, tidy mind' really resonates with us. In this chapter, we wanted to share with you some tips and techniques we've learned over the years to help keep our houses, and therefore our heads, in order. These are clearer, more concise ways to get your head around all those life obstacles and challenges so you feel more in control, and everything else seems much more manageable.

Oh, and we fully admit to not having our sh*t together all the time. There's about a fifty-fifty chance that you'll find all these techniques fully implemented at any one time, but they make us feel much better when we do.

The Clear-Out

GEMMA • First things first, clear the clutter. You can't really see what you have until you have less, and there is scientific evidence showing that having less really can impact how clearly we think. It can help with the overloaded brain feeling, as we can more effectively do what we need to do because everything is more ordered. I recently watched the documentary *The Minimalists* (on Netflix, featuring Joshua Fields Milburn and Ryan Nicodemus), which asked what would happen if you got rid of one item from your home every day for a month. Josh explained that in America, the average amount of items in one household is 300,000 – isn't that crazy? But if you break it down, that includes every book, every fork, every spoon, every pair of knickers, every sock, every piece of Lego, and so on. It really made me pause and think: what is all this 'stuff' I have, and does it bring purpose to my life?

So, I gradually started to remove the 'stuff.' Cupboard by cupboard, drawer by drawer, shelf by shelf. I found that I had so many things that either didn't work, had no function in my life now, or hadn't been used or touched in years. Do you really need twelve mismatched mugs? Or do you tend to just drink from the same mug every day? What are you keeping the rest of the mugs for? This exercise is worth a go if you feel like the clutter in your home is overwhelming, or if you feel like you have too many tabs open in your brain. Whether we realise it or not, the 'stuff' around us has both a mental and physical impact on our well-being.

Even just the thought of clearing things out can be overwhelming, so don't set a timeline for it to all be done. Deal with one shelf in your utility room while the dinner is cooking in the oven; tackle one cupboard in the kitchen while overseeing your kids doing their homework; sort the bathroom cabinet while listening to a work Zoom call that doesn't need much focus; or simply dedicate a Sunday morning to the linen cupboard while listening to a podcast. Be ruthless, and you'll be surprised by how much you can get done in a short amount of time. Better yet, you'll soon to notice a difference, and that will give you the buzz you need to carry on and get as much 'stuff' cleared out as possible. Slowly but surely, it can become a mindset.

TIM top 10: Key areas to organise

Once you've cleared out everything that you don't need, the things that make the cut need to be put away properly (just as we did with your wardrobe starting on page 103). Using drawer dividers, storage containers and a labelling system will mean that everything stays in its proper home. This makes your home easier to manage and easier to tidy up, and can help you be more time efficient. Here are a few key areas you can focus on to make your home tidier and your life simpler.

1. **Bedding:** As soon as the sheets come out of the machine and are dry, fold them into a pile depending on whose bed they belong to, rather than the type of bedding they are. Each pile should have a bottom sheet, duvet cover and pillow cases, so it can be grabbed out of the cupboard in one go when you need it. If space is a problem, pop the relevant items for each bed inside one of the pillow cases so you can stack them rather than lying them next to each other on a shelf.
2. **Towels:** One day I realised that I didn't need seventeen towels for a household of four. You only need enough towels to get you through two weeks without doing laundry. Fold bath sheets in one pile and hand towels in another.
3. **Tupperware:** Another item that people tend to hoard! Stack the lids together (left to right) at one side of the cupboard, then stack the boxes on top of each other, against the lids to hold them up. And remember, no one ever needs a crazy amount of Tupperware!
4. **Pots and pans:** Stack your pots and pans, then stick adhesive

pot lid holders (Joseph & Joseph do brilliant ones) to the back of the drawer or shelf so they don't take up much space.

5. **Bathroom cabinets:** Maximise your cabinet space by using containers, trays or boxes to separate your products into categories. Label them so you can quickly see what is where. Medicines can all be put together in one storage box and kept in a cupboard elsewhere.

6. **Cleaning products:** These can all be kept in one caddy in a cupboard. There is no need to own too many cleaning products. It's a weird thing: we all like to have loads of cleaning products, but realistically, you rarely need more than these seven items: all-purpose cleaner, disinfectant, bleach, glass and mirror cleaner, toilet cleaner and some sponges and cloths.

7. **Food tins and jars:** We usually can't actually see what food we have stored because it's all just shoved in, meaning we end up wasting money buying yet another can of sweetcorn, only to find out we already had four. Use a tiered rack for tins and spices so you can see exactly what you've got.

8. **Crackers and biscuits:** Save space by decanting all your biscuits and crackers so you have one airtight container for crackers and one for biscuits. There's no need to take up room on the shelves of your kitchen cupboards with all the packaging that comes with each individual pack.

9. **Cereals:** Same as above. Filling up my cereal containers is one of my favourite household activities. I have large plastic containers from Amazon, and each one fits about two or three packets of cereal, so it saves space (and obviously looks more aesthetically pleasing!).

10. **Entryway:** As a drop zone for everyone who comes into a home, the area around your front door can easily become cluttered and dysfunctional, getting even worse in winter as the layers build up and the shoes become chunkier. Storage space is usually at a minimum in this area. The best thing to do is add a small bench

or unit so shoes can be kept underneath or inside it, with decorative baskets on top to house those small items that so easily go missing, like keys and missed mail slips. If space allows, add some wall hooks to give coats a home.

An Eco-Friendly Home

While going through the process of organising your home, you could also think of some simple switches that can help you to become more eco-friendly. Did you know that a single plastic bottle can take up to 450 years to decompose? And over 1 million trees are destroyed daily to make toilet paper?[12]

We want to help contribute in whatever way we can to make our planet a better place for our children to grow up, so one day I decided to stop buying cling film to see how long I could go without it,* and from there I took on the side hobby of researching into simple, sustainable swaps we can make in our kitchens that have an impact on the planet with barely any effort involved. Some of these swaps can be pricey, but there are definitely more cost effective ways to be eco-friendly now than there were a few years ago. Buying in bulk can make a huge difference here, and doing this also reduces waste and means fewer trips to the supermarket, which ultimately makes your life easier and more time-efficient.

---

* Spoiler – it's been two years and I still haven't bought any!

Eco-friendly swaps

Out	In
Regular washing-up liquid	Reusable silicone squeezy bottle and Ecover Washing-up Liquid Refill
Cling film	Beeswax wraps or silicone lids
Ziplock bags	Evolve biodegradable storage bags
Synthetic washing-up sponges	byMATTER compostable cleaning cloths and Composty eco sponges
Laundry detergent pods	Smol plastic-free laundry tablets
Toilet paper in plastic packaging	Who Gives a Crap loo roll (wrapped in paper and made from 100 per cent sustainable bamboo)

Home Gadgets, Hacks and Apps

Life is hectic. Life is chaos. If you're ever sitting there, scrolling through Instagram, thinking, 'Wow, they look like they have their sh*t together,' then let us tell you now. We don't. And neither do 'they'. But there are a few things that we have come across over the years that help us take shortcuts in our days and make us feel like we have things under control.

TIM top 10: Home gadgets that make our lives easier

While some gadgets are all hype and fake promises, our curated list of gadgets have all been tried and tested, and are firm favourites in our households. These game-changers will save you time, elevate your cooking skills and help you be a more organised version of yourself.

1. **Collapsible laundry basket:** Who wants a laundry basket hanging around, taking up space? A collapsible laundry basket is the answer; when you're not using it, just fold it up and store it down the side of a cupboard or under your bed. Life changing.
2. **Beauty carousel:** Is your dressing table a riot? A rotating beauty organiser will help to keep everything in check. It's also a great way to see what you have, and can help you to avoid excess clutter.
3. **Label maker:** If you take one thing from this list, make it this. When we feel discombobulated and we don't know where to begin to get things in order, a label is a great starting point. We label everything, from the shelves in our kids' wardrobes (if they know where things go, they can help) to our food storage containers.
4. **Steamer:** Neither of us own irons, and we haven't for years – it's all about steaming! Fridja are known for their full-height vertical steamers, which are used behind the scenes at Fashion Week, but their powerful handheld version (£75) is foolproof, heats up within forty-five seconds and lasts for fourteen minutes. Another great option is the Cadrim: it heats up within twenty seconds, can steam continuously for nine minutes (enough time to get through nine items) costs just £33.
5. **Car vacuum cleaner:** Sadly, we will never be those people with pristine cars. Ours are covered in snack wrappers (kids) and empty coffee cups (us), and always sprinkled with a liberal dose of crumbs. It used to drive our husbands mad, until we each invested in a car vacuum. Who knew such a thing existed? These

USB-chargeable mini hoovers are designed to be kept in the boot of your car, and whipped out whenever you need.

6. **Salad chopper:** We want to be healthy, but sometimes healthy is boring. We want to eat delicious salads, but they never quite turn out like they do in restaurants. Well, let us introduce you to the Brieftons Quick Push Salad Chopper (£24). This absolute game-changer chops any fruit or vegetable into the most precise little cubes in seconds, with not a single bit of effort required. It makes salads easy, interesting and delicious.

7. **Shower drain catcher:** Not very sexy, but *very* useful – and your future self will thank you. Lay it over the drain in your shower, and it will collect all the hair. Then you can easily lift it out and shake it into the bin to stop your drains clogging.

8. **Multi-charging dock:** Sick of having hundreds of chargers in the kitchen for various electronic devices? These stations charge an Apple watch, ear pods and a phone all at once, all on one slick station.

9. **USB lighter:** Never hunt for a box of matches again; a rechargeable USB lighter with an elongated handle makes lighting candles (whether Diptyque or birthday cake) super-easy without singeing your fingers (or your mani!). They're also great as a stocking filler when you don't know what to buy. Every household needs one.

10. **Digital tyre inflator:** A really useful item to keep in the boot of your car. If your tyre pressure light comes on, this is so simple to use. Just undo the screw, connect the pump and press 'start'. It also has a really bright torch on it, in case you want the light for safety at night.

TIM top 10: Home hacks to make life easier

These simple cleaning and organising hacks can help you keep things running smoothly with minimal effort.

1. Want your cutlery to look super-shiny and as good as new? Scrunch up a ball of kitchen foil (about the size of a small fist) and pop it in the utensil container in your dishwasher along with your cutlery. Pop the machine on. The foil will remove scratches and water marks, and leave your cutlery sparkling clean.

2. Car windscreen frozen over but you're in a hurry? Then fill a ziplock bag (we like Evolve Together, as they are biodegradable) with warm water (not boiling, just a little warm from the tap) and swipe it over your screen. Watch the frost instantly dissolve.

3. Can't wash out medicine syringes properly? Separate the syringe and pop them in your dishwasher, placing them upright on the prongs that are used for holding up bowls.

4. Freeze wine into ice-cube trays and just grab a cube or two from the freezer when you need it for cooking, rather than having to open a new bottle.

5. Have kids? Keep a toothbrush upstairs and downstairs to save time in the mornings. Also, if you are an 'after-breakfast' brusher, you don't need to waste time going back upstairs again.

6. Line your bin with newspaper so it absorbs any juices from food.

7. Slice an old toilet paper roll down the middle and place it around wrapping paper rolls so they don't unravel.

8. Use hair straighteners to 'iron' collars and cuffs.

9. If candle wax spills on to a surface, DON'T SCRAPE IT WITH A KNIFE! Instead, pop some ice cubes into a plastic bag, lay it on the wax for a few minutes, and then you'll be able to just lift the wax off without damaging the surface.

10. Have a fancy bottle of handwash on your sink? When it runs out, refill it with a cheaper one. No one will ever know.

TIM top 10: Apps to make your life a breeze

These days, it seems that there's an app for everything. Here are ten that we couldn't live without.

1. **Keep Notes:** Run by Google, this is a great way to manage your to-do lists. You can share it with a partner (in business or life) and it syncs as you go. We have a shared TIM Keep Notes, which keeps our business running smoothly. You can make checklists that can be ticked off, or just general notes that can be organised with titles and by colour or theme.

2. **Free Prints Photobooks:** We all want to be that person that has chronological photo albums of our lives, but if you're still stuck back in the 2021 zone, you need this app. Each month, you can create a free photobook, straight from your phone.

3. **The Modern Milkman:** Picture the scene: it's 8pm and you realise that you have no milk for breakfast the next morning. Open this app, and you can have fresh milk, juice, bread or other store-cupboard essentials waiting for you come morning. From Derbyshire to Deptford, they've got you covered.

4. **Google Earth:** We pretty much get lost everywhere we go. A quick glance at Google Earth before we set off makes everything feel more familiar when we get there, because rather than just coloured squares on a map, you're seeing the real roads and houses. Trust us, it works.

5. **Flo:** Tracking periods should be a government requirement! This app makes it really simple to note down days, dates, symptoms and feelings, so that when you are feeling emotional or grumpy, are having intrusive thoughts, find yourself low on patience, or are suffering from backache (delete as applicable), then you can check the app and it will show where you are in your cycle – and probably explain why you are feeling that way.

6. **Ocado:** Having a food shop delivered to your door is a game-changer. We both have a regular slot at 7am on a Monday

morning, which eliminates the stress of finding time to get to the shops, and it means we can just add to it throughout the week when we notice we've run out of something.

7. **Shell:** No need to go into the petrol station when you are filling up. With this app, you can park at the pump, use the app to log which pump number you are at, then fill up. Just confirm on the app when you are finished and drive off. This is so useful if you have kids in the car and don't want to leave them, or if it's pouring with rain, or if it's dark and you don't feel safe going into the petrol station.

8. **Amazon:** An Amazon Prime subscription (free next-day delivery for a year) should be bought for every new mum. Need batteries tomorrow? Prime it. Need a gift for your auntie's birthday that you forgot about? Prime it. Wrapping paper? Prime it. Run out of Garnier Micellar Water? Prime it. You catch our drift!

9. **Ruuby:** Short on time? Erm, that's all of us. Ruuby is genius. We know we already mentioned this app on page 96, but it really *is* that good. Like Uber or Deliveroo but for beauty, you can 'order' the treatment you need to your door, and it's all paid for via the app. There is nothing better than having a full-body massage and then just going up the stairs to bed, without battling your way home. Available in London, Manchester and the Cotswolds, and rolling out to more cities soon.

10. **Balance:** If, like us, you are on the edge of perimenopause and menopause, then this app is for you. It was created by renowned menopause specialist and GP Dr Louise Newson, and it allows you to track your symptoms day to day, to see if there is a pattern forming. It is expert-led and full of medically approved pockets of information that will help guide you through this hard-to-navigate chapter of life.

■ ■ ■

This chapter should have given you a lot to think about. Use it as you wish: declutter as you go; work your way through the tips; take screenshots of the lists to refer back to; download the apps; add the gadgets to your Amazon baskets. You'll hopefully start to feel a little lighter. And then, all of a sudden, you'll find that things feel just a little easier.

Let us know how you get on.

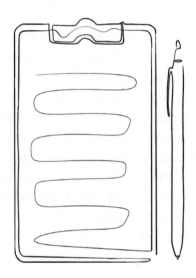

- 11 -

the TIM method in the kitchen

SAM • When we were brainstorming topics that we should cover in this book, we kept coming back to food. When we feel hugely overwhelmed and short on time, a home-cooked meal is often the first thing to go, and it's easy to find yourself swapping a warm dinner at the end of a stressful day for toast, crackers or cereal. But we feel so much better when we eat well. We are more productive, and we have more energy. As the saying goes, you can't pour from an empty cup.

We both really enjoy hosting, be it dinner with friends, family occasions or Christmas Day – which we've both been hosting for the last eight years. But one of the differences between the two of us is that I love cooking, discovering new recipes and creating dishes for my friends and family, while Gemma would quite happily never cook, ever (lucky for her, her husband is an excellent cook and really enjoys it!).

I'm all about easy entertaining. For me, the key to successful hosting is to keep it simple and streamlined. I play it safe. Never will you find me trying out a new recipe on a night when I have ten people over for dinner. I have a repertoire of recipes that always impress, but are super-simple to cook.

Whenever I throw a dinner party, and talk about it on Instagram, I'm asked to share my recipes. So here are some of my favourites. Some have been passed down through my family, and some are my own. The best bit is that they are simple, yet delicious; these recipes can either be prepped in advance the night before, or thrown together in under half an hour after a crazy day at work. I hope you, your friends and family enjoy these recipes just as much as I do.

Dinner Party Recipes

My chicken shawarma

This is my failsafe dinner-party recipe. You do all the prep the night before, so all that's left to do is put it in the oven as your guests arrive. Shawarma is a traditional Middle Eastern marinated chicken dish. I like to serve this with fresh pitta and a selection of dips and salads (tahini, hummus, aubergine dip, chopped cucumber and tomato salad – the vegetable chopper from our gadgets list on page 186 is excellent here), which means very little cooking is actually required. I've shared this recipe with so many friends, who always have huge success at their own dinner parties when they make it.

Serves 6–8

12 boneless chicken thighs
zest and juice 2 lemons
100ml olive oil
4 garlic cloves
6–8 tablespoons shawarma spice mix

- Combine all the ingredients in a large, resealable bag, and mix well to coat the chicken. Place in the fridge and leave to marinate for 6–24 hours.
- When you're ready to cook, remove from the fridge and allow to come to room temperature. Preheat the oven to 220°C/gas mark 7.
- Tip the marinated chicken thighs into a roasting tin, making sure they lie flat and are not piled on top of each other. Roast for 30 minutes.
- Cut the roasted chicken into strips and serve with your chosen accompaniments.

My great-grandma's chicken soup recipe

The nickname for this sort of traditional chicken soup is 'Jewish Penicillin' because it's the cure-all for any ailment one may have – from a cold to a broken heart. Make it, eat it, freeze it for when you need it. It's typically dropped off to a friend going through a hard time, such is its power to fix all problems. I find that it's best made the day before if you want the flavours to develop to their maximum and to get it to a golden colour. If I'm making it for Friday night dinner, I make it on a Thursday morning, leave it to cool, then refrigerate it overnight. On Friday afternoon, I'll bring it to the boil, then leave it to simmer. Delicious! This recipe was my great-grandma's, passed down to my mum, who passed it down to me – and now I'm passing it down to you ...

Serves 8

½ chicken carcass/boiling fowl from a butcher (usually no more
    than £2) – this will make the richest soup, but alternatively you
    can use a roasted chicken carcass
1 onion, quartered
2–3 large carrots, sliced
2–3 celery sticks, chopped
1 tablespoon chicken stock powder (I like Telma or Osem)
freshly ground black pepper

- Put all of the ingredients into a large pan, then fill the pan to the brim with cold water until everything is covered.
- Bring to the boil, then reduce the heat to low and simmer for about 7 hours. Taste to check the seasoning to your liking. Before serving, strain to remove the carcass.
- That is it! It's so easy, it's always a hit whenever I make it for anyone, and it really does cure all.

My best friend's crispy cauliflower

My husband Nick is a fussy guest, with food allergies and very specific requirements when it comes to his ratios of apple to crumble (this will make more sense later). Knowing this, my best friend pulls out all the stops when we go to hers for dinner. This is one dish she knows he will always rave over, asking for seconds and thirds. I find side dishes hard; they need to be interesting without being overpowering, and not too time-consuming. Her crispy cauliflower is a real table-pleaser, and looks as effort-full as it is effortless.

Serves 6–8

1 medium cauliflower, cut into florets
200g plain breadcrumbs
2 teaspoons paprika
½ tablespoon onion powder
½ tablespoon salt
½ tablespoon freshly ground black pepper
3 eggs
150ml milk
2 tablespoons chilli paste
vegetable oil spray
125g Greek yoghurt
2 teaspoons lime juice
2 tablespoons sweet chilli sauce

- Preheat the oven to 180°C/gas mark 4.
- In a small deep bowl, mix together the breadcrumbs, paprika, onion powder, salt and pepper.
- In another small bowl, beat together the eggs and 110ml of the milk. Stir in 1 tablespoon of the chilli paste.
- Dip the cauliflower florets into the egg mixture, then toss in the breadcrumbs to coat.

- Arrange on a large roasting tray and spray with vegetable oil spray. Roast for 20 minutes.
- While the cauliflower is cooking, mix the yoghurt, remaining milk, remaining tablespoon of chilli paste, lime juice and sweet chilli sauce in a small bowl.
- Serve the roasted cauliflower with the dip.

My leftover chicken pie

This is the perfect way to use up leftover chicken from a roast. I either make one big pie, or a few smaller ones in ramekin dishes that I then freeze. This pie is a great comfort food to drop off for a friend or family member in need. I tend to make this for anyone who's had a new baby, or has something going on in their lives that means they don't have the time to cook.

Serves 4

glug of olive oil
half a leftover roast chicken, or you can use chopped chicken breast
2 leeks, sliced
150g mushrooms, sliced
1 tablespoon plain flour
2 teaspoons Dijon mustard
1 tablespoon crème fraîche
300ml chicken stock
1 sheet of ready-rolled puff pastry
1 egg, beaten
cornflour (if needed to thicken)

- Heat the oil in a large pan over a medium heat. Add the chicken and warm through – if you're using raw chicken breast, cook for 3 minutes.

- Add the leeks and mushrooms and cook for 3 minutes, then stir in the flour. Now add the mustard, crème fraîche and stock, and stir well. Season with salt and pepper and leave to simmer for 5 minutes. If needed, you can add a teaspoon of cornflour to thicken.
- Preheat the oven to 200°C/gas mark 6.
- Unroll the pastry and make sure it's big enough to cover the top of the ovenproof dish you'll be using. Criss-cross the pastry with a knife.
- Tip the chicken mixture into the ovenproof dish, then lay the pastry over the top. Pinch the edges of the pastry to attach it to the dish, and add a pretty pattern or some pastry letters to the top if you're being cute. Brush all over with beaten egg.
- Bake for 15 minutes or until the pastry is golden.

My mother-in-law Jill's epic toffee apple crumble

As I mentioned earlier, Nick is exceptionally fussy when it comes to apple crumble. He once accidentally insulted my mum by suggesting her crumble-to-apple ratio was not quite perfect – and it has never been forgotten. However, his mum Jill's apple crumble *is* pretty much perfect, and it's fair to say that nothing and no one has ever bettered it. I begged her to share the recipe with me.

Serves 6–8

For the crumble
175g cold butter, cubed
350g plain flour
350g caster sugar
handful of oats
1 teaspoon cinnamon (optional)

For the apples

1½ tablespoons butter

20 small apples, peeled and chopped (Jill says she prefers not to use cooking apples)

1½ tablespoons soft dark brown sugar

1 tablespoon maple syrup

1 teaspoon amaretto (optional)

- Preheat the oven to 190°C/gas mark 5.
- To make the crumble, tip the flour into a bowl. Add the butter and rub it into the flour to form a crumb-like texture. Add the sugar, oats and cinnamon, if using, and stir. Set aside.
- For the apples, heat the butter in a large pan over a medium heat. Add the apples, along with the sugar, maple syrup and amaretto (if using). Stir gently for five minutes until the apples look slightly brownish and glistening.
- Tip the apples into an ovenproof dish and heap the crumble topping over the top. Bake for approximately 1 hour, until the top looks golden and the inside is slightly bubbling through. Cover with foil if the top starts to brown too quickly.
- Eat on the day with a dollop of custard, or freeze.

My cheat's Lotus Biscoff ice cream cake

I've been making this for years; it's such an easy one to make ahead of time and works brilliantly when you need a quick vegan recipe. All you need are three ingredients.

Serves 8

store-bought pie crust (or feel free to make your own) – choose a dairy-free one if you're making this as a vegan dish

750ml vegan vanilla ice cream (I use Swedish Glace)

400g jar of Lotus Biscoff Spread (must be the crunchy variety – not smooth)

- Allow the ice cream to soften a little, then tip it into a large mixing bowl. Add the entire jar of Biscoff spread and use a wooden spoon to mix the two together.
- Spoon the mixture into the pie case and smooth it over.
- Freeze overnight.
- That's it. When you're ready to serve, pop the cake on to a cake stand (this makes it look super-fancy) and cut into slices.

Chocolate bark

The easiest addition to an after-dinner coffee or mint tea. Break it up into pieces and serve it on a pretty dish. If you prefer, you can make this using just one type of chocolate, but I like the marble pattern achieved when using three. I switch up the toppings depending on the occasion. An effortless crowd-pleaser.

Serves up to 10

2 × 100g bars of white chocolate
2 × 100g bars of milk chocolate
2 × 100g bars of dark chocolate
toppings of your choice (raisins, dried cranberries, pistachios, chopped apricots, sprinkles – whatever you like)

- Preheat the oven to 200°C/gas mark 6 and line a baking tray with baking parchment.
- Place the chocolate bars on the prepared baking sheet in a pattern (e.g. from light to dark, or alternating). Pop this into the pre-heated oven for a few minutes to gently melt. Keep checking on it so it doesn't burn.

- Once melted, remove from the oven and use a knife to swirl the melted chocolate together in marbled patterns. Scatter over your chosen toppings.
- Freeze overnight (make sure to keep the baking sheet flat in the freezer).
- Once frozen, break up into pieces and serve.

My Weekend Go-Slow Recipes

My easy banana cake

I feel like Covid kind of ruined banana cake's rep, but I love banana cake. I've been making this one for years and it's so simple that even my kids know the recipe by heart. It's just the perfect recipe, and I love to whizz one up when we have friends coming over for afternoon tea.

Serves 6–8 (makes one medium loaf)

125g butter
200g caster sugar
2 eggs
3 ripe bananas, mashed
2 tablespoons milk
½ teaspoon bicarbonate of soda
185g self-raising flour
a few drops of vanilla essence

- Preheat the oven to 180°C/gas mark 4 and grease a medium loaf tin with butter.
- In a bowl, cream together the butter and sugar. Add the eggs one

at a time, mixing after each addition, then stir in the mashed bananas and vanilla essence.

- Add the milk, bicarbonate of soda and flour, and stir well to combine.
- Pour into the prepared tin and bake for 40 minutes.
- Allow to cool in the tin for a few minutes, then turn out onto a wire rack to cool completely.

This is Mothership's famous fluffy pancake stack

Until I hit upon this recipe in May 2020, I'd never been able to master the art of pancake-making, but now it's easy. We eat ours plain, but you can top them with anything your heart desires. This simple recipe has been brightening up TIM followers' weekends for years; it's actually one of our most viewed blog posts ever. There's a little sugar in the recipe (2 tablespoons, and it makes around 8–10 pancakes), but I don't mind this as a treat for my kids. They don't have them every day. If you'd prefer to not add sugar, maybe sweeten them up afterwards with fruit as a topping.

Makes 8–10

135g plain flour
1 teaspoon baking powder
2 tablespoons caster sugar
120ml milk
1 large egg, lightly beaten
2 tablespoons melted butter (allow to cool slightly), plus a little extra
     for cooking

- Sift the flour, baking powder and caster sugar into a large bowl. In a separate bowl, lightly whisk together the milk and egg, then whisk in the melted butter.

- Pour the milk mixture into the flour mixture and, using a fork, beat until you have a smooth batter. Let it stand for a few minutes.
- Heat a non-stick frying pan over a medium heat, and add a knob of butter. When it's melted, add a ladleful of batter. It will seem very thick, but it's meant to look like this. Wait until the top of the pancake begins to bubble, then turn it over and cook on the other side until golden brown. The pancake should be about 1cm thick.
- Repeat until all the batter is used up. Serve with whatever toppings you wish!

My mum's shakshuka

These baked eggs in a delicious tomato-based sauce make the perfect go-slow weekend morning brunch, lunch or dinner. I am obsessed: it's real Israeli-style comfort food. You can add anything you like: halloumi, sausages, everything works. Serve with warm slices of pitta, challah or toast. No one can resist it.

Serves 4

1–2 tablespoons olive oil
½ onion, finely chopped
100g cherry tomatoes, halved
1 red pepper, finely sliced
400g passata
2–4 eggs
Handful of crumbled feta
salt and freshly ground black pepper

- Heat the oil in a shallow pan over a medium heat. Add the onion, tomatoes and peppers, and cook for five minutes until softened.
- Pour in the passata and bring to the boil, then cook for about five minutes until reduced by a third. Season well.

- Make some hollows in the mixture and crack the eggs into them. Cover the pan with a lid and leave to cook for a few minutes, or until the eggs are cooked to your liking.
- Crumble the feta over the top and serve.

★ **TIM TIP:** Frozen chopped veg is your friend, as are frozen chopped onions, garlic and frozen chopped herbs. Frozen leeks are even better, because who has a leek when the recipe calls for one? M&S even do frozen individual portions of tomato pasta sauce, which you can use as a base for so many recipes – including this shakshuka. Plus, they're always useful when a kid comes over who only eats pasta and sauce. Thank us later.

For those nights when you just can't face it . . .

Because at least once a week we *do* have cereal for dinner, here are our favourite 'brinner' (breakfast for dinner) options. And yes, our kids often get brinner too – because some nights, you just need to give them something easy, filling and quick!

- My favourite is Crunchy Nut Cornflakes – usually around the time of my period, when I'm craving sugar.
- Gemma's favourite are Weetos: an oldie but goodie. With cold milk, they're just divine!
- Our other favourite brinners include toast and peanut butter, good old scrambled eggs, or a delicious bowl of porridge on a cold winter's night – always topped with cinnamon.

Cake Gate

Baking cakes for our kids seems to be something we've inadvertently become famous for. We started at their first birthday parties, thinking it would be a really cute thing to do, and now they totally expect it. With fond memories of flicking through our mums' nineties baking books, we get it. But also, now that we're the mums, when do we stop doing these kinds of things? Anyway, we always have big ideas, but they rarely (read, never!) go to plan. All our past Cake Gates are saved in our highlights on our Instagram, but if you're after some inspo, here's what we've 'created' over the last eight years . . .

Sam's Grandma Joyce's chocolate Victoria sponge

I use my Grandma Joyce's famous chocolate cake recipe as the base for all my cakes. Nothing and no one has ever beaten this. Honestly. Her cakes were iconic in Sheffield. She passed away when I was pregnant with Alfie, and I get such warm feelings, pulling out her recipe card with her neat, curly writing on it, and recreating the cake that she would have made for all my dad's birthdays, and my own.

Serves 10

For the cakes
2 teaspoons cocoa powder
175g unsalted butter, softened
175g golden caster sugar
3 medium eggs, beaten
150g self-raising flour

For the chocolate buttercream
1 teaspoon cocoa powder
85g unsalted butter, softened
175g icing sugar
a few drops of vanilla extract

- Preheat the oven to 190°C/gas mark 5 and line 2 sandwich tins with baking parchment.
- In a cup, blend the cocoa with 3 teaspoons of hot water and leave to cool.
- In a large bowl, cream together the butter and sugar until pale and fluffy. Add the cooled cocoa mix and beat until blended, then add the beaten eggs, one at a time, beating between each addition.
- Fold in half the flour and mix, then fold in the rest.
- Divide the batter between the prepared tins, levelling the surface.
- Bake both cakes on the middle shelf for 20 minutes until springy to the touch.
- Leave to cool in the tins for 5 minutes before transferring to a wire rack to cool completely.
- Meanwhile, in a large bowl, cream together the ingredients for the chocolate buttercream until smooth.
- Once the cakes are cool, sandwich together with the chocolate buttercream.

Postman Pat and his bright red Porsche

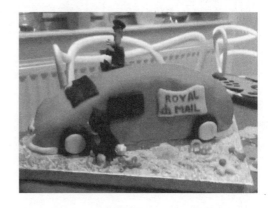

Sam's creations over the years

Postman Pat's van: It ended up so flat it looked more like a Porsche.

Fireman Sam's fire truck: I copied a BBC recipe; it was fairly easy and one of the best so far.

Mickey Mouse: A regular chocolate cake, with two smaller circular ones at the top as ears. I chucked chocolate buttons at it instead of creating a 'face'. Bit of a cop-out.

Batman cake: This one was all about black ready-to-roll icing and a Batman cookie cutter.

Ninjago cake: IYKYK. If you don't, I hope you never have to.

Swimming pool: Eight out of ten on the ease scale. Chocolate fingers around the edge are your friend.

Football pitch: Just don't use dyed green desiccated coconut for the grass – it goes *everywhere*.

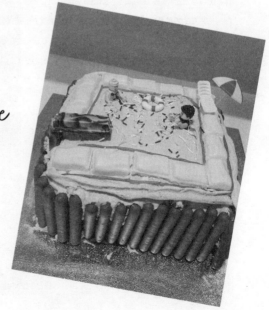

My swimming pool cake
– easy but effective!'

Gemma's creations over the years

Minnie Mouse: In theory, pretty simple, but for some reason Minnie looked like her creepy Aunty Mavis.

A beach and mermaid: I made two round cakes, stacked one on top of the other, and piped swirls of icing from bottom to top in a few shades of blue. I use crumbled-up digestives for the sand and popped a tiny mermaid doll on top. I also used a mould to make shells out of fondant, then dusted them in edible gold powder. Sounds fancy, but it was really simple to do.

Princess castle: This was for Belle's fourth birthday, and the first time I considered retiring from Cake Gate. The windows slid off (it was in the middle of a July heatwave) and the turrets looked phallic!

A farm and tractor:
The easiest one I've ever made. A rectangular sponge, some piped icing as grass, a tractor toy stolen from my Ace's toybox, a few farmyard animals and some chocolate fingers for the fence.

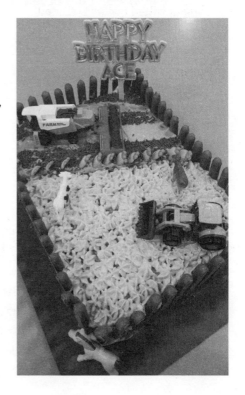

Gemma's BFF Debbie's cupcakes

My BFF Debbie is a brilliant baker. Her creations are out of this world, real works of art, and the kind of thing she could charge loads for. About eight years ago, she wrote down her recipe for simple cupcakes, and ever since I've used it when I'm baking, as it works just as well for regular cakes. My cakes rarely look pretty, but the feedback is pretty consistent: they actually taste good! I combine Debbie's recipe with a cream cheese frosting, for purely selfish reasons. I've always found buttercream icing too sickly, and find that cream cheese frosting takes the edge off. I've used this recipe for years and it always tastes good.

Makes 24 cupcakes, or a two-tiered round cake

For the cakes
250g unsalted butter, softened
2 teaspoons vanilla essence
350g caster sugar
4 eggs
375g self-raising flour
250ml milk

For the cream cheese frosting
300g unsalted butter, softened
300g icing sugar
600g full-fat cream cheese

- Preheat the oven to 180°C/gas mark 4 and line 2 sandwich tins with baking parchment, or two 12-hole cupcake tins with cupcake cases.
- In a large bowl, cream together the butter, vanilla essence and sugar. Beat in the eggs, one at a time, until well combined. Gradually stir in the flour, followed by the milk.
- Pour the batter into the prepared tins or cases.
- Bake for about 15 minutes (if it's cupcakes) or 20 minutes if you

are making the cakes, until golden and cooked through. Leave to cool in the tins for 5 minutes before transferring to a wire rack to cool completely.

- Meanwhile, make the cream cheese frosting. In a large bowl, beat the butter until soft and creamy, then add the icing sugar and cream together until you have a smooth, buttercream consistency. Now work in the cream cheese with a wooden spoon (don't beat it). If it's too runny, then leave it in the fridge for 10 minutes and it will firm up.
- Sandwich the cakes together and ice (or ice the cupcakes) with the cream cheese frosting.

Simple cake for Belle's fifth – she loved it!'

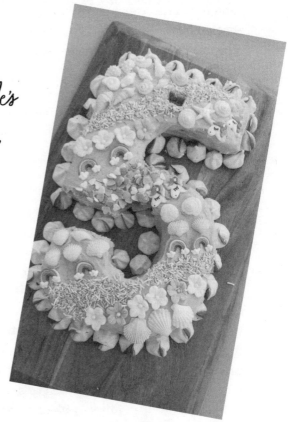

- 12 -

the TIM guide to travel

We've lost track of the conversations we've had with friends and family about where to go on holiday, and we get DMs on a weekly basis asking for our hotel recommendations.

We love to travel. Travelling to the fashion capitals of New York, Paris and Milan twice a year was a huge part of our previous professional lives (we both worked backstage at Fashion Weeks, Sam reporting on beauty and hair looks, and Gemma furiously pinning outfits and getting models lined up). These days, carving out time to spend abroad with friends and family is one of our biggest privileges and joys in life. Whether it's a long-haul trip, a UK staycay or a sneaky weekend micro-break that gets you thirty-six hours in the sunshine before landing back at your desk at 9am on Monday morning, we've now got it sussed.

Hopefully, this chapter will give you food for thought and a few new ideas, and save you a few hundred lost hours on Trip Advisor.

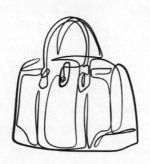

Getting There: How to Travel in Style

Packing tips

GEMMA • How often have you heard the phrase, 'Life is about the journey, not just the destination.' Not only is this brilliant life advice (!) but it's also very relevant for travelling. Planning a trip can be stressful enough, so when it comes to what you wear when actually travelling, you want it to be as stress-free and comfy as possible. As much as people say you are more likely to get a free upgrade if you dress up, that ain't happening these days! How people travel in heels is beyond me. Comfort is key, and therefore only loungewear is allowed (disclaimer: my husband is one of those crazy people who always travels in jeans!). I usually recommend travelling in a co-ord or matching set. This outfit can then be utilised on the trip and worn together or as separates, dressed up for a night out, or worn casually with sandals during the day. Go for breathable fabrics (like cotton or linen) so the air can circulate between your body and clothes. If you opt for synthetics (fabrics from the 'poly' family, like polyester, polyamide, etc.), you'll notice you get sweaty and sticky much faster.

I tend to travel in my chunkiest sandals so I don't have to pack them, and I always pop socks in my hand luggage, as there is nothing worse than cold feet on a plane.

When it comes to what bags to travel with, a backpack is easiest, as it keeps your hands completely free. If this is what you choose to take, then it can be useful to take a small cross-body bag for your essentials in the airport (phone and passport), so that you don't need to keep taking the bag off your back to retrieve them. If, like Sam, a backpack isn't your thing, then do as she does and use your beach bag. This also saves it from getting squashed into your case. Bag dividers are so useful to make it easy to grab what you need. You can use zippered pouches, pencil cases or old make-up or toiletry bags. I have one pouch for passports, documents, phone, wallet and headphones, another pouch for toiletries, another pouch for snacks, and so on.

Once your hand luggage is sorted, it's time to think about your suitcase. Obviously, this all depends on where you are going and how long for, but I have two tips that I swear by, have stuck with for years, and are relevant no matter where you are off to, or for how long.

1. Pack in outfits

Lay out your full outfits (trousers, top, shoes, jewellery, belts and underwear) in a pile so you have something there for each day. You can, of course, duplicate outfits, or mix and match certain pieces with others that you are packing. If this is the case, then write a note on a sticky note and add it to the outfit pile. This way, you won't forget anything. You don't necessarily need to pack your clothes into the case in their outfits, although this might make it easier when it comes to unpacking, as you can take them from the case and put them directly into your wardrobe when you arrive on your trip.

2. Use packing cubes

I'm not quite sure how I ever got through life without these! Whether you pack in outfits or not, packing cubes are so useful and can make the unpacking process much more time-efficient. If I'm packing for myself, I tend to pop all my outfits in the case, then I put all my undies in one packing cube, my accessories in another and my swimwear in another. Then I add my toilet bags. When you arrive, you can just lift the cubes from the case to a drawer or shelf, unzip and leave it all in there. It also makes unpacking so much easier. There's no need to carry loads of piles from suitcase to washing machine – just pop all the dirty laundry into cubes (one for lights, one for darks) and carry them to the wash. You can get more durable cubes that are made from thicker fabrics with really sturdy zips (I love my Tiba & Marl cubes; I've owned them for years and they've come on so many trips), or you can get cheap and cheerful ones that will still do the job but may not last as long as their sturdier counterparts.

Once you've sorted your outfits and got your cubes, I would always recommend rolling rather than folding. This is a tip I learned from my Grandma Ann. Rolling your clothes means they won't crease as much, and you can squash more into the nooks and crannies of your case.

In-flight beauty essentials

SAM • We all want that post-holiday tell-tale golden tan to show off when we land back on UK soil, but do you find you return home with a few unwanted skincare souvenirs too? Dry, flaky skin and pesky breakouts put a dampener on that après-sun glow. When you combine the high altitude, increased UV exposure and recirculated air of an airplane, it can be a recipe for a complexion disaster.

Your pre-flight checklist should include more than just your boarding pass and carry-on – how you prep your skin before you set off is just as important. From inside-out hydration to packing layers in your hand luggage, here's how to land looking – and feeling – totally refreshed.

Prepare for take-off

When I say take-off, I'm talking about taking off the make-up. Those in the know never travel with a full face (I'll explain why in a moment). If you can't bear to make it through the airport without anything on your skin, make sure you pack a mini bottle of micellar water and some reusable cotton pads into your hand luggage so you can remove everything once you get settled on the plane. Don't forget to anti-bac those hands first.

My in-flight kit

Mist: Clinique offer a 30ml version of their famous Moisture Surge Face Spray (£8.40). This refreshing, fine mist has the most subtle scent, so is great for quenching thirsty skin in enclosed spaces. Spritz a few times mid-flight. Ignore the looks.

Serum: Byoma Hydrating Serum (£12.99) is a 30ml bottle full of clever ingredients that increase the skin's hydration levels *and* prevent moisture loss. Refillable, too – clever.

Mask: Sheet masks were the golden child of the beauty world until we all woke up and realised that single-use products were not the best for the planet. Skin Republic is an Australian brand selling sheet masks made of a compostable cupro fibre, which breaks down in just ten days, while the packaging is also fully biodegradable and breaks down in around thirty-two days. I like their Hyaluronic and Collagen Sheet Mask (£3.74).

Lip balm: I'm not fussy here. Good old Vaseline or Carmex sticks do the job, although it is a good idea to invest in one that also offers SPF50. Ultra Violette, Beauty Pie and Ultrasun all have great options, depending on your budget.

Rehydration station

You lose up to 30 per cent of the skin's moisture after a four-hour flight. Plane cabins are pressurised to simulate conditions found at 7,000 feet – the equivalent of being on top of a mountain – which means less blood and fewer nutrients are transported to the surface of your skin.

Your body loses roughly one cup of water for every hour you're in the sky. Drink as much water as you can get through while in the air. Moisture is also pulled from the skin as the humidity drops, leaving it super-thirsty. This can lead to oily skin, breakouts and puffiness. This is where skincare layering comes in. I swear by anything containing hyaluronic acid when I fly. As we learned on page 20, it can hold up to 1,000 times its own weight in water, and binds hydration to the skin. Layer this with occlusives and emollients (like ceramides, which create a barrier that lock in hydration). See page 23 for a list of our favourite ceramides.

Once you're in the air, layer up: you need a mist, a serum and a sheet mask. Masks are the best way to hydrate the skin intensely during a long-haul flight. It decreases water evaporation, meaning that the hydrating ingredients are better absorbed. Leave it on for the recommended fifteen to twenty minutes, then massage any residue into your skin. And don't forget your lip balm (a stick not a pot if we're being fussy – hello, germs!).

Battle puffiness

Air pressure combined with fluid retention from salty in-flight snacks and sitting for long periods create the perfect storm when it comes to making your face look puffy. In-flight plane food is loaded with salt, and unless you're my husband, who *loves* plane food, you'd probably be happy to give it a miss and swap it for fruit or a sandwich from Pret and a bit of facial massage instead.

Using a hydrating serum or facial oil, sweep your hands from your chin to the bottoms of your ears, and then down to the collarbone. Repeat a few times to flush away excess fluid. Now, use the same sweeping motion from your cheeks to your ears and down to the collarbone. And repeat.

Prepare for landing

Flying during the day? SPF is just as important while you're in the air as it is on land. In fact, UV radiation levels are twice as high at 30,000 feet (the altitude of most commercial flights) as they are at ground level. Finish off your in-flight routine with a layer of SPF, and hop off the plane with flawless skin when you touch down on the tarmac.

Touchdown: Beauty essentials for when you reach your destination

Here are our favourite holiday partners, for face and body.

Face

As we explained on page 25, we must start our days with a two-finger dose of SPF. Sun damage creates some of the most visible signs of ageing and, more importantly, puts you at risk of melanoma.

La Roche-Posay Anthelios Age Correct SPF50+, £25

This is not just an SPF; this ground-breaking, anti-ageing factor 50 contains a cocktail of active ingredients to protect your skin for the future. Hyaluronic acid hydrates skin as it basks in the heat, while niacinamide brightens dark spots. And forget the SPF of old that used to cause breakouts; here, LHA acids dissolve clogged pores, leaving your skin blemish free. It's super-lightweight, and doesn't leave a white cast on dark skin tones. Perfect as a make-up base.

CeraVe AM Facial Moisturising Lotion SPF50, £14

A fast-absorbing SPF50 that can be used instead of your daily moisturiser. Powered by CeraVe's patented delivery system, MVE technology, moisturising ingredients are continuously released throughout the day; ideal in a hot climate. It also helps protect the skin against pollution particles. Developed with dermatologists, it's suitable for both normal to dry, and acne-prone skin. It leaves no white cast, so works on all skin tones. It's TikTok famous for a reason.

Ultra Violette SPF50 Re-application Mist, £32

That first layer of sunscreen is a no-brainer, but reapplication is the bane of my existence. We know that SPF protection doesn't last all day; this is why SPF top-up sprays are your BFF. This spray is absolutely phenomenal; the nozzle is so well made that it emits the finest mist that sits so nicely over make-up, adding a glow. In my mind, it's one of the best and most sophisticated out there.

Garnier Ambre Solaire Over Make-Up UV Protection Mist SPF50, £8
Not everyone has £32 to spend on an SPF spray, so this is a brilliant second best. Pop it in your handbag, and reapply over make-up when needed.

Body

SPFs have come a long way from the sticky, staining products of the past. These days, applying a body SPF is much more of a luxurious moment, treating the skin as well as protecting it. You'll be excited to actually use them.

Garnier Ambre Solaire Eco Designed Protection Lotion SPF50, £7
If you were blind-testing SPFs, you would have no idea that this was under £10. With broad-spectrum UVA and UVB protection against immediate and long-term skin damage, the formula is so silky it's a dream to apply, leaving skin feeling soft and hydrated. It also smells like a super-luxe hotel lobby, and its science is backed by the British Skincare Foundation. The bottles are made with 100 per cent recycled plastic and are fully recyclable.

Vichy Capital Soleil Solar Protective Water SPF50 Enhanced Tan, £20.00
Every beauty editor's best-kept secret. A clear water formula enriched with high-protection UV filters and natural beta-carotene to help a deeper, longer-lasting tan form safely. We have never burned while using it. Super-lightweight and quickly absorbed, it's a genuine joy to apply – and it doesn't stain your clothes.

Our Little Black Book of Travel Destinations

We get asked questions about our holidays on an almost daily basis. We both like to travel, and we were never scared of travelling when our kids were tiny babies. We've been on some fabulous family holidays together and apart – we have different criteria when it comes to holidays. Here, we've shared some of our favourite destinations, whatever your travel style.

The micro-break

Sometimes you just need to step outside of your life for a hot second. Do you feel like you're drowning in work/life admin, being pulled in a million different directions and dealing with constant brain fog? If so, a micro-break is exactly what you need. Ideal for when you're feeling over-worked, over-stressed and over-screened. A micro-break is for when you don't think you have the time to go on a mini-break, or you don't want to (or can't) get away from work/pets/kids (delete as appropriate) for very long. The key to a micro-break is to find the shortest flight possible that will allow for maximum relaxation time at your destination. Sometimes you just need to press the reset button. We're calling it; micro-breaks are the new mini-breaks, and there is something to suit all budgets.

The romantic one: Paris

SAM • The trick with a micro-break is to choose somewhere that only takes a few hours to get to, and take the earliest mode of transport to get there. When we were drowning in early parental life, Nick and I escaped for a one-night micro-break to Paris. The first Eurostar of the day left St Pancras at 7am, getting us into Paris in time for a 10am croissant *petit dejeuner*. We stayed in the **Hoxton Hotel**. The location was perfect (a fifteen-minute walk to the Louvre), the food was fabulous, the beds were super-comfy and the service was epic. It wasn't too pricey either, at £250 a night. A day of sight-seeing and walking later – my top tip is to get a legendary takeaway hot chocolate from the Parisian institution **Angelina** and then walk through the Tuileries – the 4pm Eurostar the next day got us back to London just in time to put the kids to bed.

The girly one: Amsterdam

GEMMA • My sister lived in Amsterdam for a couple of years, and after we discovered how easy it was to get to, we ended up visiting often. The flight from London is just over an hour, and the train from the airport to the city centre is just fifteen minutes, so it's perfect for a forty-eight-hour micro-break. Get an OV Chip Card (similar to an Oyster card) if you are planning on getting trams or cycling everywhere, which is a great way to travel around; otherwise, cabs are easy. There is so much to do, but just wandering through the charming streets along the canals is beautiful. Our favourite place to eat was **Food Hallen**, a huge food market where great food meets a brilliant atmosphere. Don't miss out the museum quarter, which is situated beside PC Hooftstraat (similar to Bond Street). Jordaan is a beautiful place to wander, with independent shops and cute cafés. No trip to Amsterdam is complete without visiting the Anne Frank House. Stay at **The Conservatorium** (worth stopping for a drink, even if you don't stay), **The Pulitzer**, **Volkshotel** or **Sweets Hotel**.

The party one: Saint-Tropez

SAM • What I am about to tell you will blow your mind. It's possible to spend forty-eight hours in Saint-Tropez, get a tan and have an epic night out without taking a day off work. At £70 per person, a 7am Saturday flight from Heathrow got us to Nice for 10am, and we arrived at the legendary **Byblos Hotel** just in time for a late breakfast in the courtyard. Five minutes' walk away are all the big names – Celine, Fendi and Chanel – while Chloé, Valentino and Vuitton line the square by the Gendarmerie. Walk a little further towards the port, and the cobbled streets are lined with independent boutiques selling brands like Paloma Blue and Hunza G. The market is held on Tuesdays and Saturdays, and the straw basket game is strong. As the sun drops, head down to the port to watch the sunset with a cold glass of rosé at **Le Girelier** before dinner at **Le Quai** (French–Asian cuisine; the tuna sashimi is great). Book a table outside to yacht-watch and be ready for the best cabaret you'll see on the Riviera. Le Quai turns into a club and is open until 3am.

The next day, we headed to **Le Club 55** for more rosé, seafood and steamed artichoke. A legendary beach club institution (book well ahead and wear your best bikini), it's a free ten-minute shuttle from Byblos, who waved us off with beach towels in a canvas bag. The crudité platter is famous (less of a platter, more of a farmers' market on a plate), and the party vibe is ten out of ten. One 9.40pm flight later, and you'll be in an Uber home by 11pm, refreshed, relaxed and ready for the week ahead.

The staycation

'Staycation' is an American term, defined in the *Cambridge Dictionary* as 'a vacation that you take near your home, rather than travelling to another country'. We all fell for staycations during the Covid years (bookings surged 300 per cent in the summer of 2021) and it's safe to say that the UK is more than equipped for an in-country holiday.

It's worth noting that staycations aren't always the cheap option. But when you don't want to – or can't – fly, perhaps because you are travelling with a dog, have a family occasion to celebrate or prefer to do more than 'fly and flop' on vacation, it's a great shout. Staycations also support the local economy, reduce your carbon footprint and let you skip the jetlag. Take the stress out – and free up space in the car – by booking a food delivery slot ahead of your arrival.

We are both big fans of family staycations, and have rounded up a few favourites we've been on over the years.

The one by the sea: Cabu, Kent

Just under two hours outside of London lies a little slice of coastal heaven. Composed of a dozen different-sized self-catering wooden cabins nestled amongst the wildflowers on the edge of the Kent coast, Cabu opened in 2019 – the chicest thing to happen along the English Channel – while Cabu Cotswolds opens summer 2024.

Cabu is cleverly done; there are chic interiors, speedy Wi-Fi and fresh Gail's pastries to satisfy city-dwellers, but you still feel remote and removed from the hectic pace of daily life. It's like Soho Farmhouse – before it became too bougie and far removed from the real countryside – but with a £180-a-night price tag. The relaxed vibe just makes you instantly at ease.

Accommodation
There are two- and three-bed cabins. A two-bed cabin is perfect for a family of four. It consisted of a master bedroom with the comfiest, cosiest bed and floor-to-ceiling windows looking out on to the bay (but with brilliant blackout curtains), and a second bedroom with bunkbeds, and enough space for a wooden cot should you need one.

The lounge is roomy and the sofas are ridiculously comfy. At night, we lay and watched the sun set through the Crittall windows with the log fire lit. All the furniture was from Loaf Home and John Lewis, with Soak and Sleep pillows, striped robes and Dr Bronner's eco toiletries.

Details
An outdoor heated pool, communal BBQ area and being just a stone's throw to St Mary's bay make this the ideal outdoorsy getaway. The promenade is great for bike riding. Dog friendly.

The one in the countryside: The Grove, Hertfordshire

Whenever anyone asks us to recommend a really special staycation, we always answer, 'The Grove.' There is something so incredible about this place, which opened over twenty years ago. Every time we visit is just as special as the last. Of course, we are lucky that we live just twenty minutes away. This has meant that The Grove has become our special place: it's where Nick first told Sam he loved her; it's where Gemma found out she was pregnant with Belle; it's been the site of friends' weddings; and, as This is Mothership, we've hosted some amazing events here.

Accommodation

There are two options: the eighteenth-century Manor House and the more modern Main Hotel. We'd say that the Manor House is slightly fancier, but the rooms in the hotel are roomy and newer, with a foldout sofa bed, perfect for a family. When it comes to food, there's so much choice. Our favourites are the Glasshouse, a luxury all-you-can-eat 'buffet' full of various five-star international food stations, and Madhu's at The Grove for all the Saturday-night vibes, alongside mouth-watering South Indian cuisine.

Details

The Grove is set in the most beautiful grounds, which are incredibly versatile. Visit in summer and you'll find an Everyman outdoor cinema and a 'beach', complete with open-air swimming pool (and spectacular kids' club). Visit in autumn, as the leaves fall, and you'll find an outdoor music trail and treasure hunt set up for kids. Over Christmas, their table of events includes outdoor burger stations, craft tables and soft-play set-ups. In the school holidays, they host Football Escapes at The Grove. And, of course, the famous golf course and award-winning spa are givens.

The one near Gemma's home town: Gleneagles

Gleneagles is like heaven on earth. When you go up the driveway to this beautiful Scottish hotel and spa near Auchterader, you feel like you are being transported to a different world. Inhaling the pure Scottish air is enough to calm down even the most stressed person, and spending a couple of days in this haven can zen you out more than you would ever think possible. Just an hour from Glasgow or Edinburgh airports, it's easy enough to escape to for a couple of nights. Gleneagles isn't modern, but it's utterly charming and luxurious, without being pretentious.

Accommodation
This place is perfect with children and without, as it accommodates both options in equal measures. The rooms are as cosy as can be, with sumptuous velvet sofas, beds comfy enough for a princess, views for miles and, best of all, free movies. We lost count of the restaurants (we think we counted seven), which serve everything from bar snacks to brasserie food.

Details
Perfect for those after outdoorsy pursuits; whether you're teeing off, climbing trees, taking aim, or going horse riding – you can do it all here. But if you'd rather snuggle up indoors and hide from the Scottish weather, then the spa is where you need to go! The kids' club is also one of the best I've ever been to.

The one for a large group: Temple Guiting

Long before Soho Farmhouse, Daylesford and the Beckhams moved in, Temple Guiting sat in the heart of the Cotswolds. Embodying the quintessentially English idyll, the estate consists of the main Tudor manor house, which sits next to the refurbished, more contemporary-looking stables and barns.

Accommodation

Hire the whole estate, which sleeps thirty, or select just one or two of the accommodations for smaller groups. Onsite, you'll find a secret cinema with a full library of movies, an outdoor pool, hot tubs, a tennis court, a children's playground and a rowing lake for wild swimming (if that's your thing). Inside, the accommodation is fully stocked with all mod cons: Dyson hairdryers, Nespresso coffee machines and iPod docks (just BYO food; it is self-catering). It has the royal seal of approval too; King Charles is a big fan of the immaculate gardens.

Details

Located half an hour from Cheltenham, it's very easy to reach by car, train or plane. The Wild Rabbit, the Plough Inn and the Hollow Bottom pubs are only a short drive away. Visit Daylesford Organic nearby – check out their roster of events, as there's often something fun happening – or swing by Bicester Village on your way home.

The ones in Central London

If you want to splash out: Claridge's, Mayfair

If budget allows, or it's a big blowout birthday, then Claridge's cannot be beaten. There is something so special about this place: from the second you step through the door, you are treated like royalty, but it doesn't feel pretentious. We've both taken friends and family here for birthday breakfasts, and every guest – whether staying or eating – is treated in the same warm manner. They are also fully welcoming of kids.

If you're heading to the West End: The Hoxton, Holborn

Ideally situated in the heart of theatreland, we really rate The Hoxton in Holborn. A cosy room starts from £200 a night, the location is amazing (walking distance to Covent Garden, Soho, Leicester Square and Oxford Street), plus it's doggy-friendly and family friendly, and has a yummy restaurant open for everything from breakfast through to late-night snacks.

If you are on a budget: The Pilgrm, Paddington

A reasonably priced hotel, in a brilliant location, The Pilgrm has a certain charm about it, with parquet floors that date back 200 years, combined with modern touches. Ask for a room on the side if you want it to be a bit quieter. The rooms are small and the staff are friendly; if you need a bed for the night, this is a good option. Rooms from £139.

The vacation

Deciding where to go on holiday can take months of research. There's so much to consider when choosing a destination, including flight time, time difference and cost of flights. And when you finally settle on somewhere, pinning down the perfect hotel can take even longer.

We both like totally different types of holidays. Sam loves the three Cs – chill-out, childcare and cocktails – while Gemma isn't a fan of sunbathing and prefers a bit more exploration (with a side of beach, of course!).

Here, you'll find a selection of our favourite destinations, but they're not just hotel recommendations. As we get older, our desire to see the world and immerse ourselves in culture is getting stronger (gah, we're turning into our parents), so you'll also find our favourite restaurants, markets, beaches and places to explore within each country. And if anyone has an itinerary for the perfect West Coast US trip, then please send it our way.

Mallorca

GEMMA • Way back in 1987, my parents, together with my aunt and uncle, bought a two-bedroom flat on the south-west coast of Mallorca, and so I've been lucky enough to visit Mallorca every year since I was three years old. It's my happy place. I got married there in 2010, I brought my daughter there when she was eight weeks old, and it's where my son learned to swim. It's a two-hour flight from London, with just a one-hour time difference, so it's a really accessible and easy place to holiday. You have guaranteed sunshine from April to September, although I've been before in October and it was 30°C.

We've travelled all over the island, eaten in plenty of the restaurants and swum at so many of the beautiful beaches. The food is delicious, and the sand and sea at some of the beaches can rival the Maldives. The island has such a lovely, relaxed vibe; no need for fancy outfits or your high heels (unless you really want to!).

Accommodation

Hotels are in abundance on the island, with something to suit all budgets. My advice is to stay on the coast. Inland is beautiful, but being able to see and walk to the sea, especially during the peak summer sun and heat, makes such a difference. **Cap Rocat** is a beautiful hotel that used to be an ancient fortress, and is one of the most exquisite locations I've ever seen. They have three restaurants. **The Mardavall** is super-pricey but super-fabulous, plus they have an exceptional kids' club. **Hotel Migjorn** has been rated as one of the best family friendly hotels in Spain; it's a rural finca in the south of the island, near one of the most beautiful beaches Mallorca has to offer, Es Trenc (which has lots of sightings of pink flamingos in the summer months!). The **Melia Alcudia** is similar, but a bit more basic. The rooms have all that you need, and are very spacious. The pool can be bedlam in high summer, and has no shallow end (although there is a small standing-only kids' pool). The huge beach of Alcudia is just a three-minute walk away, with the whitest sand and the bluest sea you can imagine.

Eating

You can find restaurants to suit every budget here. There are some super-special places if you want to splash out, as well as plenty of really casual, reasonably priced restaurants on the beach that have a great atmosphere. **Lume & Co** is more inland, in quite a secluded location, but it's such a pretty setting and has gorgeous food. Great for dinner. **S'esponja** is one of my favourite little nooks in Mallorca: a tiny restaurant right at the edge of Calvia beach. Book a table on the dock right on the sea for an adults-only romantic night, or up on the decking if you are going with kids. **Cappucinos** is a Spanish chain of restaurants. Our favourite one is located in Puerto Portals. Make sure you sit outside at the front, as you'll have a great view of all the super-yachts that come into the port, and it makes for excellent people-watching. **Mar Y Mar** is at the back of the beach in Peguera. Try to book a table at the front so you are overlooking the sea. Great for cooling down over lunch, or for dinner. **Illeta at Camp De Mar** is located on a tiny island just off Camp De Mar beach; walk along a wooden bridge over the sea to access it. Book a table on the water's edge – and promise me you'll jump into the sea from the rocks after. They have a kids' menu, clean toilets (with an exceptional view) and the restaurant is buggy-friendly.

Beaches

Alcudia Beach is a huge beach, with every type of water sport, loads of sun loungers and a walkway over the sea that is just crying out to be jumped off! Soft, white sand and crystal-clear water. **Cap Falco** is a tiny but perfectly formed cove. Park at the top of the steps and walk down (there are a lot!) or drive down a dirt track on to the beach for free parking. It has one small but excellent café (you must book to get a table) and very few sun loungers, so if you want one, you need to be there early. **Camp De Mar** is a tiny beach, with shallow waters and a wonderful restaurant (Illeta, mentioned above). There is a free car park nearby. **Peguera Beach** is huge, with the most epic waves at all times (I'm not sure how or why, but the waves are always *so* big there!!). It has lovely soft sand, and a pirate-themed assault course for kids, which is great when you've all had enough sun. See above for Mar Y Mar restaurant, which is a must if you visit this beach. The beach right at the end of the infamous port **Puerto Portals** is wonderful. The port can sometimes be a bit pretentious, but the beach is anything but. It has a small café at the back, and paddleboarding for €9 an hour. Clear sea, white sands.

Dubai

SAM • I think Dubai gets a bad rap. To be honest, it never appealed to me, until we used an expiring BA Companion Voucher on a whim in December 2018. We've returned five times since.

There are so many hotels, so it can be hard to narrow down where to go. Price is obviously the most important factor, but you should also consider location, facilities and *vibe*. Do you want calm and serenity? Do you want more of a party feel? Do you need places to walk to within the resort, or would you be happy getting cabs to restaurants? Dubai has something for everyone.

Accommodation

The Jumeirah strip is one big private beach resort with five hotels set around the Madinat. You can use whichever beach, swim in whichever pool, and eat in whichever restaurants you want. It just comes down to which hotel you prefer, what you need, and your budget (each hotel differs in price and offers different facilities). We love **Jumeirah al Naseem**; as a family, we are (currently) very happy to all sleep in one room on holiday, keeping costs down. The beauty with the rooms in the al Naseem is that they have sliding doors, separating the lounge area (and the sofa bed where the kids sleep) from the bedroom, meaning you can zone off the room if you need to. The bathrooms are also huge, and the wardrobe space is plentiful – something that is often a squeeze when fitting four people into a room. We have also stayed twice at the **Four Seasons**. The hotel is beautiful, the service is faultless and the facilities are absolutely stunning. In terms of restaurants, you have all the fancy ones there – Nusr-Et, Scalini, Coya – making it a great grown-up option. As my kids got bigger and needed more space, we looked for other hotels with more facilities, like water parks and football pitches, etc. That's when we discovered Jumeirah al Naseem.

Eating
Food can be pricey in Dubai; the equivalent of London prices. At the Jumeirah al Naseem, children under four eat free, which is invaluable when it comes to ordering lunches and snacks from the pool bar. The half-board dine-around option is amazing for adults; with over forty restaurants between the hotels, you have so much choice that you never need to leave. From noodle bars and high-end sushi to steak houses and Thai, Mexican and Chinese restaurants, there are so many choices. The majority of them are covered by half-board, but for some you may need to pay a supplement.

Details
The Wild Wadi Waterpark is included in a stay at any of the Jumeirah hotels, and residents get free daily access. To get around Dubai, we either use Uber or the Careem app, and drivers always have car seats in the boot (pristine, obvs). We use Black Lane for airplane transfers. The Sonara Desert Experience is a must: go sand-surfing and camel riding, play beach football as the sun sets, then enjoy a five-star theatrical dinner experience under the stars (kids can watch a movie on beanbags).

Cyprus

SAM • Beautiful in the summer, Cyprus is also an ideal destination for some autumn sunshine. This is one of the few places in the Med where summer weather clings on well into late October. The island of Cyprus is one of the largest in the Mediterranean, and a recent revamp has seen many new hotels pop up. Five hours from the UK, cheap flights are abundant, so the hard part is choosing where to stay.

Accommodation
We stumbled upon **Parklane Hotel** in Limassol in 2021, and have been back three times since. In fact, Nick will kill me when he realises that

I've given the details away, but in terms of cost (we book the cheapest room, approximately £290 a night for four in a double room, as the only time we are there is to sleep), as a luxury five-star hotel with top-class facilities – three pools, a shopping village, world-class restaurants and a beach with sea that stays warm well into November – it's hard to beat. Of course, Limassol's seafront is lined with gorgeous hotels; you may want to look at the **Four Seasons** and the **Amara** too. On the Paphos side, the **Almyra** and its sister hotel the **Annabelle** are both brilliant for families and adults-only trips alike.

Eating

The food at the Parklane Hotel is pricey (**Nammos** and **LPM** are the in-house restaurants) but Limassol marina and old town are a ten-minute taxi ride away, and the castle area is lined with gorgeous places to eat. I love the **Uptown Square** collection of outdoor restaurants, which is a ten-minute walk away.

Details

There is so much to see and do in Cyprus, if you can make it off the sun lounger. The Tombs of the Kings and the Blue Lagoon trip to see the Baths of Aphrodite grotto top my list.

Marrakesh

GEMMA • My ideal holiday is some sunshine (hot but not too hot), culture (it's important that my kids understand how diverse our world is) and excellent shopping. Marrakesh ticks all the boxes. I visited for the first time with eleven members of my family in April 2022, and it won my heart. There is so much to soak up: the culture, the customs, the colours, the food, the souks, the smells, the kindest people, the interiors and the architecture.

Accommodation

We stayed at **The Fairmont**. It has the largest pool in Marrakesh, beautiful grounds, kind staff and an excellent kids' club, and is not at all pretentious.

Eating

We ate in some incredible restaurants, but the ones that came up trumps were **Plus 61** and **Nomad**. Plus61 is run by Australian expats. The fried chicken starter was immense, as was the lemon tart. Nomad overlooks the Medina, so make sure you ask for a table on the roof for the best view. We sat there while listening to the call to prayer, and the atmosphere was amazing.

Details

You can't visit Marrakesh without wandering through the souks. The main square is called Jemaa Elf-Na, and if you walk through this square it leads you down small, narrow alleys that all lead into one another and are like Aladdin's caves. They sell everything from clothes to jewellery, to pottery. Would you believe me if I told you I bought a sink?! A beautiful monochrome black and white tiled sink for £40. Brought it home as hand luggage – EasyJet weren't best pleased!

We went with children aged two to six, and initially it was a pretty big culture shock, but by the end of day one they were so immersed, as there is so much to look at and so many different things to see. It can get really busy in the markets, so we held hands through those parts, then they could roam when it got quieter.

Something that really stood out to us was how totally spotless everywhere was. The markets were pristine, and there was no litter anywhere. We chatted to the market stall owners and heard stories of where the pieces were made and how the stalls had been in families for years and years, and it was all so fascinating.

Step outside of your comfort zone: The ski trip (Valmorel)

As two avid lovers of sunny summer holidays, we did something very left-field in February 2020 and booked our families on a ski holiday. At the time, we each had a four-year-old and a two-year-old, so when the idea first came up, our initial thoughts were mixed. Our husbands (both die-hard skiers) would LOVE it, but the logistics with the kids would be a nightmare – oh, and Sam had never skied, and Gemma had last skied twenty years ago. Therefore, surely we would both rather lie on a beach than spend our holiday doing a sport, in cold weather (we don't like sports and we don't like cold weather.) But still, we went for it.

Accommodation

We stayed at **Club Med Valmorel**. We flew with Jet2 from Stansted to Grenoble, then it was a two-hour transfer to Valmorel. We fully surprised ourselves and loved it: the fresh mountain air, doing something daily that got our hearts racing, the kids' club, the unlimited food and drink, the sunshine, the hot chocolates overlooking Mont Blanc, the fact that you need to focus on what your feet are doing so you can't think about menial life tasks like laundry and after-school club schedules . . .

The skiing

We both started in beginner lessons, and our husbands went off on their own adventures. By day two, it had all come back to Gemma so she went out with the boys, and Sam stayed in the lessons all week to build confidence and learn techniques. By day three, she'd skied down a proper mountain herself.

What we wore

For the skiing part, you'll need an appropriate ski suit, or trousers and jacket, along with a couple of thermal tops, thermal leggings and thermal socks (we found Marks & Spencer thermals the warmest for us and the kids). You'll also need a neck warmer, ski goggles (sunglasses won't do because the wind and snow will get in your eyes), and proper ski gloves. For *après-ski* we were in leggings and jumpers with snow boots every night. Boots need to be warm and have a good grip.

■ ■ ■

Our travel over the years has changed slightly, as we went from being young, single and carefree to being parents of young kids, but the goals have remained the same: to immerse ourselves in the culture of different places, to educate our kids on the privilege we have in being able to travel, and to see as much as we can without spending an absolute fortune (while getting a tan, of course).

There is so much we still want to do, including road trips through Europe, driving holidays along the West Coast of America, a trip to the Philippines, and beach-hopping in Thailand. It's all on our to-do lists. We must remember to make that vision board!

If you take anything away from this chapter, we hope that it's to try new things, and not to follow the crowd. Those trips where you try something different often end up being the most memorable ones, for all the right reasons.

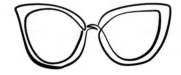

our final words . . .

If you take anything from this book at all, we hope it's that the smallest of things can make the biggest difference, whether that's an organised drawer, an outfit planned out the night before, good skin, a confidence-boosting lipstick, a twenty-four-hour break from reality. Simple tweaks, shifts and the ways you view things can move mountains. Start small, and take your time.

Thank you for reading this book, and for coming on this journey with us. We hope it's been a useful, practical and enjoyable ride. We are just two girls who met on Instagram, felt that there was a space out there for us to share our combined experiences and expertise, and somehow ended up here, adding 'author' to our bios. To write this book has been an actual dream come true, and we can't thank you enough for buying it.

Please let us know your thoughts – @thisismothership – and tag us in any photos or any words that resonate with you.

Glossary

Beauty

AHA (Alpha Hydroxy Acids) Naturally occurring acids. Lactic acid and glycolic acid are both commonly used AHAs that gently exfoliate the surface of the skin and are used to improve the appearance of skin, treating signs of ageing such as fine lines, scarring, pigmentation. Best for dryer skins.

BHA (Beta Hydroxy Acids) Used to resurface the skin as well as purging inside the pores. Salicylic acid is commonly used to treat blemishes, reducing redness and inflammation, as well as smoothing skin's texture. Best for oily, combination skins.

Humectant An ingredient that binds hydration to the skin.

Emollient An ingredient that creates a barrier.

Skin barrier The outer layer of skin that protects us from external 'threats' such as infections and allergens. When it is strong, skin is healthy.

Serum A skincare product you can apply to your skin after cleansing but before moisturising, with the intent of delivering powerful ingredients directly to the skin. Traditionally water-based.

Oil These go on top of the moisturiser because they have a bigger molecule. They're supposed to keep the creams and everything underneath moist during the entire day.

Active In skincare, active ingredients are the powerhouse ingredients that actually do the work, targeting specific skincare concerns. The more potent these are, the higher up they will be on the ingredients list.

Antioxidants These help protect skins cells from damage and ageing caused by free radicals and environmental aggressors like UV and pollution.

Free radicals Unstable molecules that damage skin cells. Caused by pollution, smoking, chemicals, etc.

Contour A technique for sculpting the face, playing with shadow and light by adding make-up that is darker or lighter than your natural skin tone.

Silicone In cosmetics, silicone makes the surface of the skin smooth and gives a 'hydrated' effect, but it can build up on skin and cause acne.

Sulphates The main cleansing ingredient in a shampoo, and what creates the lather.

Fashion

Chunky boot A boot with a large or heavy sole.

Delicate boot A slim-fitting boot in a thin leather with the ankle shaft fitting closely to your leg.

Slimline trainer A trainer that is more delicate and slim in shape, usually in a more retro style (such as Adidas Sambas, Adidas Gazelles, Vans, Converse).

Chunky trainers A trainer that has a more exaggerated, broader shape, giving it a more solid appearance (such as New Balance 530 or 9060, Nike Air Max, Asics Gel 1130).

Loafers A flat shoe that can be slipped on and off with no laces or buckles.

Proportions The dimensions or balance of a shape.

Silhouette The overall outline of a shape.

Sustainable Something that has been made in a way that causes little or no damage to the environment.

Natural fabrics Fabrics that are made from natural materials like plants, animals or minerals.

Synthetic fabrics Fabrics that are formed via chemical processes.

Care label guide

WASHING

Washing

Machine wash
permanent press

Machine wash
gentle or delicate

Do not wash

Wash at or
below 30 °C

Wash at or
below 40 °C

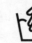
Wash at or
below 50 °C

Wash at or
below 60 °C

Hand wash

CHEMICAL CLEANING

Professional cleaning

Dry clean, hydrocarbon
solvent only (HCS)

Gentle cleaning
with hydrocarbon
solvents

Very gentle cleaning
with hydrocarbon
solvents

Dry clean,
tetrachloroethylene
(PCE) only

Gentle cleaning
with PCE

Very gentle
cleaning with PCE

Do not dry clean

WET CLEANING

Professional wet
cleaning

Gentle wet cleaning

Very gentle
wet cleaning

Do not wet clean

BLEACHING

Bleaching allowed
for both chlorine and
non-chlorine
bleach

Bleaching with
chlorine allowed
(obsolete)

Non-chlorine bleach
when needed

Do not bleach

Do not bleach

NATURAL DRYING

Drying symbol

Line dry

Dry flat

Drip dry

Dry in the shade

Line dry in the shade

Dry flat in the shade

Drip dry in the shade

TUMBLE DRYING

Tumble drying symbol

Tumble drying
(low temperature)

Tumble drying
(normal)

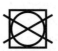

Do not tumble dry

IRONING

Ironing

Iron at low
temperature

Iron at medium
temperature

Iron at high
temperature

Don not iron

Don not steam

References

1   The research was presented at the International Investigative Dermatology meeting in 2013 and featured in a press release from Estée Lauder https://www.elcompanies.com/en/news-and-media/newsroom/press-releases/2013/7-23-2013

2   Community x SEEN Beauty Survey, the participants of which were 447 UK-based beauty enthusiasts aged thirty-plus. The research was carried out in 2023 for the This is Mothership website.

3   Danziger, Pamela, 'With recession threatening, the Lipstick Effect kicks in and lipstick sales rise', *Forbes*, 1 June 2022. www.forbes.com/sites/pamdanziger/2022/06/01/with-inflation-rising-the-lipstick-effect-kicks-in-and-lipstick-sales-rise/?sh=502843441276.

4   McKinsey & Co., 'The beauty market in 2023: A special state of fashion report', *McKinsey & Co*, 22 May 2023. www.mckinsey.com/industries/retail/our-insights/the-beauty-market-in-2023-a-special-state-of-fashion-report/.

5   Community x SEEN Beauty Survey, as above.

6   Ibid.

7   MacNaught, Stacey, 'Burnout statistics UK – job related', *Micro Biz Mag*, 21 February 2023. www.microbizmag.co.uk/burnout-statistics-uk.

8   Saad, Lydia, Agrawal, Sangeeta and Wigert, Ben, 'Gender gap in worker burnout widened amid the pandemic', *Gallup*, 27 December 2021. www.gallup.com/workplace/358349/gender-gap-worker-burnout-widened-amid-pandemic.aspx.

9   The Community X SEEN Beauty Survey, as above.

10   ONS, 'Average height and weight by age in the UK', *Office for National Statistics*, 21 June 2022. https://www.ons.gov.uk/aboutus/transparencyandgovernance/freedomofinformationfoi/averageheightandweightbyageintheuk

11   Attril, Martin, et al., 'Red shirt colour is associated with long-term team success in English football', *Journal of Sports Sciences*, 28:6, 2008, pp. 577–82.

12   Who Gives a Crap, 'Are 1 million trees really cut down each day to make toilet paper?'. *Who Gives a Crap*, July 2023. support.whogivesacrap.org/hc/en-au/articles/20748392368537-Are-1-million-trees-really-cut-down-each-day-to-make-toilet-paper-

Acknowledgements

For their expertise and inspiration, kindness and common sense, we would like to thank Sophie and Kim, our incredibly loyal talent managers at River Talent, who have been with us through thick and thin for the last seven years. Lucy and Jenny, for being so incredibly patient & helping us handle the load. And Lily, for being so efficient, chilled and organised – hopefully a little of it will rub off on us.

For making this book a joy to work on, our editor Zoe Bohm and Little, Brown. Zoe came to us five years ago and asked us to write a book, and we never got around to sending her a book proposal. Covid, two babies and four years passed, and when we finally sent it, she championed us the whole way. Thank you, Zoe.

To our followers. When we decided to set up the This is Mothership Instagram account in March 2016, we had not a single clue where it would take us. Some of you have been with us for the full eight years; some of you joined us along the way. But each of you is so important. Everything we do, everything we write, every brand we work with, we consider you first. We hope you like this book. And we hope that you find modern-day life a little easier after reading these pages. Thank you for everything that you have given us.

From Sam

For shaping my destiny without us even realising: my mum, Wendy. Growing up in her beauty salons, I absorbed so much more than either of us ever realised. Witnessing the effect that beauty can have on how women feel – not just how they look – from such an early age had such a huge effect on the journey I took, both professionally and personally. My biggest cheerleader to this day, my proofreader and my saviour, who will drop everything and take a two-hour train journey just to give me a few hours of 'me time' when I most need it. I definitely don't say it enough, but thank you, and I appreciate you.

Nick. We are not ones for mushy, gushy dedications and we much prefer bants (that'll be the Northern in us) but I have to thank you. You really stepped up here, holding the fort for hours at a time at weekends while I hid in the back of cafés with my laptop, putting the kids to bed while I panic-wrote this book into our evenings, putting up with being ignored (I'm sure you were probably quite happy watching YouTube videos about cars without me), and providing endless snacks while I was 'in the zone,' (although I'm sure RJ told you to). I love you, I love you.

Dad, for teaching me RTQ, and to always check if it can be bought cheaper elsewhere – it got me this far in life.

Jill and Steven, for all the multiple journeys up and down the motorway to babysit at the drop of a hat when I have a work event to go to. It's always appreciated. And for the crumbles, chilli, sticky toffs, and endless DIY help.

The siblings: Dan, Liv, Char, Dave. Your excitement about this kept me going one week before our deadline (five weeks into the summer holidays – whose clever idea was that?) when I really had no more words left to write.

Jo, Alix and Lisa, the three women who had a profound effect on my career, who believed in me when I didn't, thank you for all the knowledge and nurturing – and for trusting a twenty-something with big dreams and an encyclopaedic brain full of knowledge with the pages of your magazine. And for all the advice, both professional and personal.

There are numerous friends who have stepped in and helped in so many ways over the years so that I can work, taking my kids in the school holidays so that I could carve out a block of time to write, collecting them from school when I'm running late from meetings, looking after Alfie in the dark, cold, wet evenings while I watch Leo play football, or herding them at the gate (8.20am crew) so I can run to get the early train to a meeting. It takes a village, especially when you don't live near grandparents, and I am so lucky to have you all. You know who you are.

And last but by no means least, my babies. Everything I do is for you. Every late night I work, every job I accept. I chose to walk away from my dream career for you, so that I could pick you up from school every day, and that led me here. So thank you. I love how excited you are that you will be able to see this book in a real-life bookshop, and I can't wait for you to read this in the back. L and A – I love you to the squoon.

From Gemma

Please bear with me while I go into full Oscar-speech mode! I wouldn't be me without a very special bunch of people in my life, and it's very rare that I get the chance to publicly acknowledge them, so I'm going to milk it while I can!

To my Breegs: the one who knows me more than even I know me. We met when we were seventeen and have grown up together into who we are. You're more calm with a little fire, I'm more fire with a little calm, and it's the perfect combination. Thank you for understanding the importance of balance in our marriage, our household, our parenting and what we watch on Netflix. I simply couldn't do life without you, and your exceptional cheesy pasta à la Breegs.

To Susu: the matriarch, the one who taught me compassion, kindness and the importance of having a really good cleaner. Little did we know at the time, as you dragged me and my sisters around car boot sales in the rain and we moaned about being cold, drinking those very watery hot chocolates, that it would somehow shape my career today. We speak 100 times a day and it still isn't enough, and I panic if you don't know every detail of what is going on. I think there are lots of people out there who know exactly how special you are, but I don't think you realise it yourself. Hopefully you do now.

To Pom Pom: since I was twelve years old, you have phoned me at 6pm every single night, and you still do to this day, almost twenty-six years later. We have the same conversations daily –'How are you?' 'Good, you?' 'Good' – and the conversation usually only lasts a few moments, but I don't think he's ever realised how much I love these calls. He will forever be the person I ring if something really serious happens, and his advice is usually the same: 'Calm down Puds, calm down.' Love you, Dad.

To Louisa and Rachel: you are like my extra limbs, and I would be lost without you. We spend so much time together, yet it's never enough. I am so lucky that my babies have such special aunties and that we've gone on this whole journey of life together.

To my girlfriends, and especially to Dawn, Sasha, Debbie and Kerri. Thank you for understanding the importance of friendship even when we don't see or speak to each other as often as I wish we could. To my school-mum friends – Anna, Aisha and Elisha – our daily six-minute chats at drop-off and pick-up are what keep me going through each day. And to talented David M, for saving the day!

To my in-laws, for accepting early on, circa 20 years ago, that I'll never be the kinda girl who will have a hot meal on the table when you turn up at my house. Luckily my MIL is an excellent cook so I don't need to be!

To Belle and Ace: the lights of my life. My sidekicks and my soul. Thank you for understanding when I told you a million times that I was almost finished writing, and just needed another hour, and then another hour, and then just ten more minutes. I literally can't wait to see your faces when we walk into a bookshop and see this book, and you see your names in it. I will be forever grateful to you for making me a mum: my proudest achievement in life.